Orsina wrote:
I go deeper with each of her books to root out old programming and stretch my life open for new good stuff.

Amazon customer wrote:
Even though I've been using EFT for 10+ years, Tessa Cason still manages to add more nuances to the process to show me how effective and versatile EFT is. I go deeper with each of her books to root out old programming and stretch my life open for new good stuff.

A. P. wrote:
Effective and easy. This is a great self help book, much like having your own coach but more convenient and less expense. The author is very insightful, bringing positive shifts in a very short time.

Pedro Henriquez A wrote:
Tessa Cason offers us an excellent book, very practical and easy to read. The chapters on beliefs and the introduction to EFT are very clearly explained. And the different routines, very useful.

Michelle wrote:
Effective as a treatment. It works and it personalizes your issue. It takes you through a personalized process to achieve an outcome. Very effective and empowering. This is a great modality for self healing and explained in a very simple way.

Kim M wrote: WOW.

I've read several books on EFT tapping and have tapped along with various led tapping sessions and recordings. Not one thing ever changed AT ALL. I was very skeptical and couldn't understand why so many people were so sold on EFT and raved how amazingly it had worked for them and I was getting NOTHING out of it at all.

Recently after I experienced several tremendous losses within a short period of time, I was not able to deal with the overwhelming and debilitating grief. My doctor raved about EFT and strongly recommended I learn how to tap and to start now, IMMEDIATELY.

Somehow while browsing on Amazon, I found this GEM. This little book has made ALL the difference. Now I understand what it is, why it works and best of all HOW to make it work for me. The author gives an issue that everyone needs to tap on before anything else...and darned if she wasn't right. That cleared and opened a lot for me.

I am absolutely going to be purchasing more of her work on specific issues and I really feel that I am finally going to heal these issues on a deep and profound level. I wish I had found this book years ago. I will be forever grateful to the author.

Tapping looks weird, seems weird, feels weird and it's hard to believe that it really works...but yes...it works. I am just getting started with EFT and am very hopeful.

One of the very best purchases I have EVER made.

New book releases are free the first 24 hours. To know of new releases and dates for **free** downloads, please subscribe at www.TessaCason.com

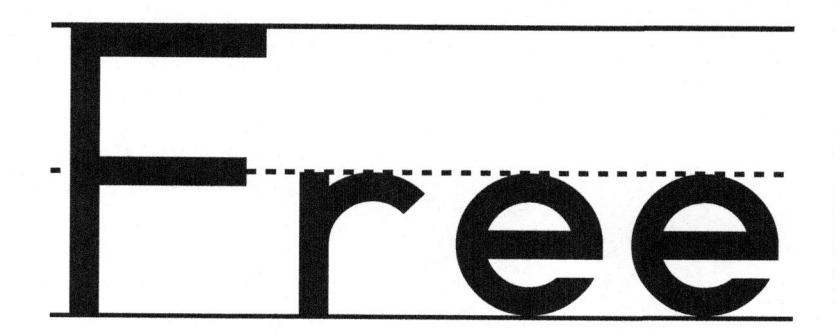

300 EFT Tapping Statements™ for Self-defeating Behaviors, Victim, Self-pity

Tessa Cason, MA

Tessa Cason
5694 Mission Ctr. Rd. #602-213
San Diego, CA. 92108
www.TessaCason.com
Tessa@TessaCason.com

LEGAL NOTICE AND DISCLAIMER:

Table of Contents

My EFT Tapping Story

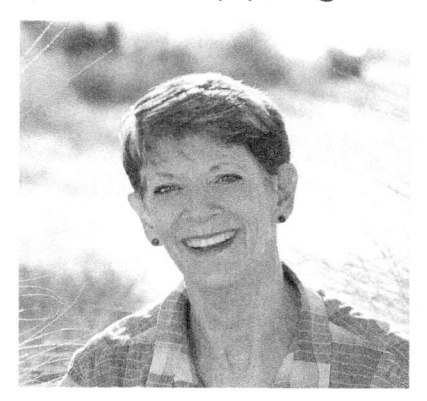

I watched from the audience as the musical group, The 5th Dimension, sang their song, "Age of Aquarius, Let the Sunshine In." In 1970, this song soared to the top of the charts. *Age of Aquarius,* I thought. *What does that mean?*

In 1970, I couldn't do a Google search for "Age of Aquarius." There weren't any websites or blogs I could read to find information about the "dawning of a new age." There weren't any YouTube videos to watch. The internet didn't exist in 1970. We had books, audiobooks on cassette tapes, and occasionally, a live, in-person seminar.

Another "new age" seeker, Cindy, and I searched for self-help, self-improvement, spiritual, and personal development classes, books, audiobooks, basically anything that could increase our awareness of the new age that was dawning.

Cindy was friends with a woman named Donna Eden. Donna had just returned from a workshop about energy. When we asked if she would teach us what was taught in the workshop, she agreed. One afternoon, a small group of us sat on her living room floor as Donna conducted her own mini workshop for us. Part of our mini workshop included how to muscle-test, a technique used to ask the body questions that bypass the conscious mind.

"Cindy, have you heard of a woman named Louise Hay?" I asked. "She is leading a workshop in La Jolla to help those with AIDS." Cindy and I attended. Louise believed that our thoughts influenced our health. In the 1970s, people didn't believe the food they ate impacted their health. The concept that our thoughts could impact our health was revolutionary for the time!

Knowing I was searching for answers on how to heal my dysfunctional childhood, Cindy suggested the "Fischer-Hoffman Process, Getting a Loving Divorce from Mom and Dad." She had just completed the program. Cindy neglected to mention the time-consuming homework, about thirty hours, every weekend for thirteen weeks! I did complete the exhausting, but liberating program.

The facilitators for the process hosted a weekly gathering in their home for Siddha Yoga and guru Swami Muktananda, the father of Siddha Yoga. After completing the program, I flew to New York and drove to the Catskills in upstate New York. I lived in the ashram for two months taking classes about Siddha Yoga, the self, and self-realization. Muktananda was in residence for a month while I was there. I attended his nightly meeting.

My journey for personal growth led to Murrieta Hot Springs in Southern California. A group called *Alive Polarity* offered workshops to transform the self. Students lived at the retreat while attending their workshops. I completed two workshops, living at the retreat for fourteen weeks. We met six days a week, six to seven hours each day. It was as intense as going through boot camp.

I learned the value of Gestalt therapy and the "empty chair technique." Gestalt therapy is a form of psychotherapy that views each individual as a blend of the mind, emotions, body, and soul with unique experiences and realities. The "empty chair technique" is used to address unresolved issues, conflicts, and emotions.

In 1985, a new breakfast group was formed called The Inside Edge. We met once a week at 6 AM for breakfast and a speaker. I heard new authors such as Brian Tracy, Jack Canfield, Mark Victor Hansen, Susan Jeffers, and many others after they had written their first books.

At this time, I was employed at The Learning Annex, assisting with hosting events. The Learning Annex was an education company that offered a wide range of classes with diverse topics. This is a short list of speakers I heard speak:

* Wayne Dyer
* James Redfield
* Dan Millman
* David Hawkins
* Deepak Chopra
* Marianne Williamson
* Melody Beattie

* Neale Donald Walsch
* Byron Katie
* Don Miguel Ruiz
* Richard Bach

In 1988, I attended a promo event for a new speaker on the lecture circuit, Tony Robbins. I returned for the weekend event, which included a firewalk. Without the internet in 1988, there were no YouTube videos or internet searches to prepare oneself for Tony or for walking on fire. Saying that *UPW, Unleash the Power Within*, was the most transformational event I have ever completed falls short of how spectacular and life changing UPW was.

The three-day event began on Friday. Throughout the first day, Tony had us do various exercises to prepare us for the firewalk. Around midnight, he marched the entire room of people to the parking lot.

As we approached the asphalt, we heard tribal drums beating, the crackling of logs burning, and smelled the burning embers. When the huge pile of wood came into view, we felt the blast of heat coming off the fire. Flames and sparks were shooting high into the air. The immediate thought one has is *Really? I am going to walk across that? That's fire. It's hot and it burns!*

Around 3 AM, everyone in the ballroom once again marched to the parking lot. We found rows of embers, ten feet long, with staff at each line. With the drums beating, excitement in the air, and everyone chanting, we lined up behind a row of coals.

When we reached the front of the line, a staff member determined if we were truly ready. They looked us in the eye, assessed our psychological readiness, looked at our body language, and told us to either go or to get back in line because we were not ready.

At the end of the bed of coals, our feet were sprayed with cool water, and then someone was there to celebrate with us. It was an amazing experience. Thirty-five years later, I still remember walking across red-hot coals and feeling triumphant as I celebrated the achievement.

In 1988, I completed every program and event Tony had, which included Date with Destiny and Mastery University. After attending all the programs, I volunteered to staff his events and helped with a dozen fire walks.

At Mastery Universe, Tony had a thirty-five-foot firewalk along with the ten-foot bed of coals. After confidently walking the ten-foot bed of coals, I walked the thirty-five-foot, and then went back and did the ten-foot bed of coals again. It was fun!

After attending numerous trainings, and earning various certificates and degrees, I established a life coaching practice in 1996, when life coaching was in its infancy. After several years, I realized that desire, exploration, and awareness did not equate to change and transformation for my clients.

Exploring the underlying cause of their pain, knowing their motivation to change, and defining who they wanted to become, did not create the changes in their lives they desired.

My livelihood depended on the success of my clients. I realized I needed a tool, technique, or method to aid my clients in their quest for change.

At the time, I knew that everything in our lives, all of our thoughts and feelings, choices and decisions, habits and experiences, actions and reactions, were the result of our beliefs.

I knew that the beliefs were "stored" in our subconscious mind.

I knew to transform and change our lives, we needed to heal the underlying unhealthy, dysfunctional beliefs on the subconscious level. I needed a tool, technique, or method to eliminate and heal the unhealthy beliefs stored in the subconscious mind.

I visited a friend who managed a bookstore and told her of my dilemma, that I needed something to help my clients truly change and transform their lives. She reached for a book on the counter near the register. "People have been raving about this book on EFT, Emotional Freedom Technique. Try it and see if it can help your clients."

In the 1990s, the internet was not an everyday part of our lives. Popular books sold more by word of mouth than by any other means. Managing a bookstore, my friend knew what worked and what did not work. I trusted my friend, so I purchased the book.

As I read the book and discovered that EFT was tapping our heads, I was unsure if this was the technique that would help my clients. I had some adventurous and forgiving clients whom I taught how to tap. When **every single client** returned for their next appointment and shared how different their lives had been that week because of tapping, I took notice! I was intrigued.

I learned that the first statement we needed to tap was: "It's not okay or safe for my life to change."

I learned that clearing an emotional memory was different from clearing beliefs.

I learned that for EFT Tapping to work, we needed to find the underlying cause of an issue.

Have you heard the joke about the drunk looking for his keys under a street lamp? A policeman asks the man what he is looking for. "My keys," says the drunk. The policeman joins in the search. Not finding the keys, the policeman asks the drunk if this is where he lost his keys.

"No, I lost them in the park."

Confused, the policeman says, "Why are you looking here and not over there?"

The drunk answers, "The light is brighter here."

EFT Tapping is a simple, yet highly effective tool to heal our issues by addressing the cause and not just the symptoms. Addressing the symptoms would be like looking for the keys under the street light. The symptoms are easily identified. But, healing the symptoms does not heal the underlying cause.

I learned we are complex, complicated beings wrapped up with a lot of history, traumas, dramas, and experiences. Sometimes finding the cause is like walking through a maze...there are a lot of dead ends, turns, and wandering around aimlessly.

Clients started asking for tapping homework. I wrote out statements for them to tap. Soon, I had a library of tapping statements on different emotional issues.

I have been an EFT Practitioner since 2000. Working with hundreds of clients, one-on-one, I learned how to successfully utilize EFT so my clients could grow and transform their lives.

Chapter 1
Introduction

Blame game, paralysis analysis, and avoidance are examples of self defeating behaviors. These behaviors have a tendency to destroy one's confidence, personal power, and self esteem.

* The victim is powerless.
* The perfectionist and people pleaser are exhausted.
* The shoulder of the martyr is sore from carrying their cross.
* The couch potato is getting fat from lack of exercise.
* The know-it-all is confused why no one wants to be their friend.

Self defeating behaviors and habits can change. It's not as difficult as you think once you light a fire underneath you and decide confidence, competence, and tenacity are qualities you prefer.

Life is a constant stream of not-so-fun stuff that will inevitably happen. We are human and our first response will be emotionally...anger, hurt, regret, shame... That's normal. What isn't normal is a repetitive pattern of thoughts, feelings, and/or behaviors that negatively impact our choices, actions, and, ultimately, our lives.

Self-defeating behaviors take us away from our goals, from what we want, leaving us feeling exhausted, disempowered, and defeated. Self-defeating thoughts are the negative thoughts we have about ourselves and/or the world around us, such as "I'm not good enough," "I have to be perfect to be accepted."

Most likely, these behaviors and thoughts have been with us most, if not all, of our lives. They might be patterns we inherited from one or both of our parents. They could be coping and/or survival mechanisms we needed to cope and survive our childhood.

Most likely, you have tried to change the self-defeating and self-sabotage behaviors, yet here you are with the same pattern. To change, we must recognize, acknowledge, and take ownership of that which we want to change.

All of our thoughts, feelings, choices, decisions, and experiences are the result of our beliefs.

To heal the self-defeating and self-sabotaging thoughts and behaviors, we need to heal the beliefs that result in the self-defeating behaviors and thoughts.

Light does not struggle with darkness when the light is turned on

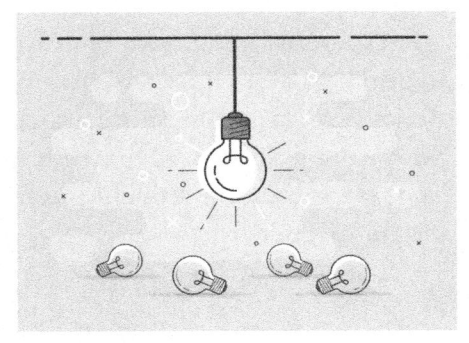

Chapter 2
Tom's Story

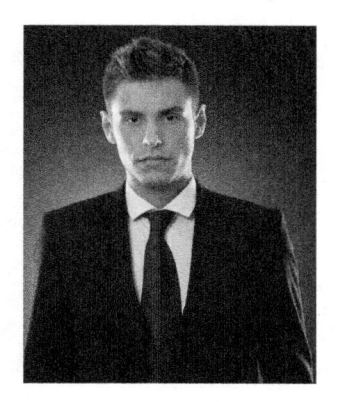

As Robert and Sam finish up their Saturday morning run, Robert asks Sam if he would work with one of his employees. The store would pay for the sessions.

"He must be a mighty important employee if you're paying my fee. You've never paid for anyone to do sessions before. This is a first!" says Sam. "Who is this employee?"

Robert slows down to a walk. Sam walks alongside Robert to the grassy field. Sitting on the cement picnic table, Robert McGregor, owner of McGregor's Department Store, says, "His name is Tom. He's a good kid. Twenty-two years old. He's worked at the store for a couple of years now."

"What seems to be the issue?" asks Sam.

"He lacks confidence, Sam. He has lots of excuses and reasons, instead of results and assertiveness. When he's late for work, it's either that he just missed the bus, or the alarm did not go off. He has a lot of talent yet never steps up to the plate to demonstrate the talent that he has," says Robert.

Sam asks, "Have you said anything to Tom about working with a life coach? Working with me?"

Shaking his head from side to side, Robert replies, "No, not yet. I wanted to talk to you first."

"What's the outcome that you hope to see?" asks an intrigued Sam.

"He has potential, Sam. I want to see him succeed. I don't think anyone has ever believed in him. I do. I do believe in him. I know that you can help him give up the reasons, believe in himself, and possibly become a great success."

Pondering, Sam says, "So, you want Tom to give up the reasons and work toward results, believe in himself, and become a great success."

Laughing, Robert says, "So you do listen!"

Sam replies, "To every word."

Remembering back, Sam asks, "Robert, I remember the day that your dad opened the store. We were ten years old, and he took the two of us on a tour before the grand opening. In the break room for the employees, he had a sign about reasons and results. Is the sign still there?"

Robert quotes the sign, "We can have the results that we say we want, or we can have all the reasons why we cannot have them. We cannot have both. Reasons or results. –Susan Carlson."

"Yup, that one."

Smiling, Robert responds, "Yes, Sam. The sign is still there. That sign is thirty-five years old."

"I think that's one of the things I remember most about your dad. I don't think I ever told you this. During our senior year of high school, I didn't know if I was going to college. Your dad had me stop by the store and offered to pay for my college education," says Sam.

Interested, Robert comments, "I didn't know that dad offered to pay for your college education. I knew that if you didn't get a scholarship, you would not have been able to go."

"I told your dad that I didn't have the grades or the money, and I wasn't sure if I was smart enough to make it through college." Thinking back, Sam starts smiling.

"Let me guess, dad gave you one of his 'Reasons or Results' speeches!"

"Yup! He took me into the break room and asked me to read the sign out loud. I was thankful that no one else was in the break room at the time. I was both embarrassed and grateful that someone cared about my future!" Robert says with a sigh.

"I don't think dad wanted to see his son's star receiver not on the other end of the football that I would throw."

Smiling, Sam says, "That too. He was mighty proud of you being a star quarterback in high school and college."

"Now you are making me feel old. We graduated from college twenty-three years ago and high school, geez, twenty-seven years ago." Hopping off the picnic table, Robert starts walking like he is a hundred years old. "I don't know if I can make it to my car without your help."

As they head to their cars, Robert asks when he wants Tom to begin. Robert responds, "What's your schedule like early mornings? I'll have Tom come see you before he starts work."

"I have some time this Friday if that works for you."

Later that day, when Tom arrives at the store, Robert asks him to come to his office. Once Tom sits down, Robert asks him if he knows what he wants to do with his life. A little surprised, Tom tells Mr. McGregor that he has never thought about what he wants. Robert asks if he has thought about the future. Tom responds that he doesn't think about the future.

Robert tells Tom about his college roommate, Sam Anderson, who is a life coach, and how he would like Tom to do some sessions with Sam to see if Sam can help him plan out a future. "Friday before coming to the store, you have a session scheduled with Sam—Mr. Anderson. His office is just down the street. The store will pay for the sessions."

Tom doesn't know if he should be offended or feel honored. No one has ever paid any attention to him... past, present, or to his future. He is a little embarrassed and not sure how to respond.

Robert writes the time and date on Sam's business card and hands it to Tom. Still a little confused and unsure of what is expected of him, Tom asks, "Mr. McGregor, the store is going to pay for my life coaching sessions?"

"Yes, Tom."

"Am I going to get fired? Is Mr. Anderson going to tell me that I'm fired?" asks a concerned, unhappy Tom.

Realizing that Tom is confused, Robert adds, "Sam is a life coach who might be able to help you figure out the direction that you want to go with your life and remove any blocks that might prevent you from creating that future."

Tom thinks about what Mr. McGregor said. "Creating a future." Is that even possible? Life happens to us. We have no choice. Well, maybe other people have a choice. Tom certainly doesn't have any choice. Even though he is an adult now, he still lives at home. His mom expects him to "contribute" the majority of his paycheck to pay for the privilege of remaining in the house. He has no choice but to work and contribute his earnings to pay his way.

On Friday, a nervous Tom sits in Sam's waiting room at the appointed time. As soon as Mr. Anderson's office door opens, Tom stands up.

"You must be Tom," says a jovial Sam.

"Yes, I am. Mr. McGregor said I had an appointment with you this morning," says Tom with some nervousness in his voice.

"Yes, you do. Come on in. Have a seat on the couch," Sam says, as he steps aside to allow Tom to enter.

After both of them are seated, Tom asks, "Am I being fired? Is that why I'm here? Did Mr. McGregor ask you to fire me?"

Laughing out loud, Sam asks, "Is that why you think you are here? To be fired? I assure you that Robert would have fired you if he wanted to fire you."

Tom lets out a heavy sigh. He realizes that he has been holding his breath ever since Mr. McGregor told him of his appointment with Mr. Anderson.

"Well, that's a heavy sigh. Relief, I guess, not to get fired, huh?" asks Sam.

"I didn't know what to think. Mr. McGregor asked me if I knew what I wanted in the future, then told me to come here. I thought that I was in trouble for not knowing what I wanted in the future. I didn't know that I was supposed to know," says Tom.

Understanding Tom's confusion, Sam says, "Let me clarify. Mr. McGregor believes in you. He wants you to believe in yourself. He wants me to help you identify what you want in the future, then remove any of the stumbling blocks in the way of creating that future."

Tom sits dumbfounded, unsure of what to say or think.

"Tom, you seem to still be confused," observes Sam.

"No. Well, yes. Mr. McGregor believes in me?"

"Yes, that's why he is willing to pay for you to do sessions with me," responds Sam.

"Mr. Anderson, I don't know how to create a future. Doesn't it just happen?" asks Tom.

"Yes. It does happen, and we can influence the direction our lives take. The decisions we make and the choices we follow through all influence the direction of our lives," responds Sam.

"Mr. Anderson, I don't feel like I have ever had a choice. I'm twenty-two years old. When I was in high school, my mom said I had to work to help support the family. My dad worked at a supermarket, and I was hired there to work part-time while I was in high school. Once I graduated from high school, my mom expected me to work full-time at the supermarket, which I did."

"How did you end up at McGregor's Department Store?" asks Sam.

"About four years ago, a friend told me about the job opening at McGregor's. I applied and felt very fortunate to be hired. I know that I haven't always been the best employee, but I really like my job and want to continue working there," says Tom.

"So, I am assuming you never went to college," comments Sam.

"No. Neither of my parents went to college. It was expected of me to work full-time as soon as I graduated from high school to help support my parents."

"Is it just you? Do you have any siblings?"

"I was the 'accident' that happened to my parents when they were in high school. My mom used to joke that she got pregnant when she didn't want to, but when she did want to, she couldn't. She really wanted a daughter. She didn't want a son."

Hearing the last comment, Sam knows that this will be a topic to return to later. Tom thinks of himself as an 'accident' and unwanted. Not a great way for a small child to be raised.

By the end of the session, Sam agrees with Robert that Tom is a great kid and needs someone to believe in him. Sam asks Tom if he would like to continue doing sessions. With a smile, Tom responds that he would. Sam asks if Friday mornings would be a good time to meet. Tom says that it is.

As Tom walks down the street to the store, he reviews the session in his mind. Mr. Anderson asked if I like my job. I told him that I do. He asked if I wanted to continue working at the store. I told him that I do. He asked what I wanted to be when I grew up, back when I was still a small child. What did I tell people when they asked? I told him that no one asked. He was surprised that my parents never asked what I wanted to be when I grew up. Huh.

Dad works at a supermarket and mom is a stay-at-home mom. Always have been. Mom says it is the responsibility of the men in the house to work and bring home their paychecks to her. It is her responsibility to pay the bills and make sure meals are on the table each day.

Mr. Anderson asked if it was enjoyable to live with my parents. "Not really," I told him. "I spend most of my time at home in my room."

He asked if I get along with my parents. "Well, I like my dad," I said. "We love watching sports together. Mom, not so much."

He asked how my parents get along. I told him the truth. He said that he wouldn't be talking to Mr. McGregor, so I felt comfortable being honest with him. When he asked how my parents get along, I told him that my mom rags on my dad, saying that he could have been someone in the supermarket. He should have been a manager, or at least an assistant manager. She tells my dad that he isn't ambitious. When she yells at him that he is a failure, only providing the minimum for his family, I go to my room.

Mr. Anderson asked what happens when I go to my room. Does mom get upset with me too? "She does," I said. "After yelling at dad, I become the next target. She comes into my room and tells me that I am just like my father and will never amount to much."

Mr. Anderson asked if I had ever thought about moving out. I guess that I haven't.

"Why haven't I thought of moving out?" thinks Tom, as he walks back to the store. Some of my friends from high school went off to school. They don't live at home anymore, except when they come home for the holidays and summer. Some of my friends who did not go off to college are still living at home.

In the days following his session with Mr. Anderson, Tom thinks about what he wants. Does he have choices? If so, what are his choices? He doesn't mention to anyone in the store that he is seeing a life coach, nor does Mr. McGregor ask him about the session. Even if someone did ask Tom about the session, he isn't sure what he would say.

The following Friday, Tom actually shows up early for his appointment. He has lots of questions for Mr. Anderson.

"Good morning, Tom," Mr. Anderson says, as he greets Tom and invites him into his office.

"How has this last week been, Tom?" asks Sam.

"Fine, I guess," answers Tom.

"Have you thought about our last session at all?" Sam inquires.

"Yes, I have," responds Tom.

"What have you thought about?" Sam asks.

"Well..." Tom starts and then stops. Looking down at his hands, he doesn't know how to answer the question. He wants to say something profound but can't think of anything. He doesn't want to come across as stupid, something his mom calls him all the time. He wants to feel worthy of Mr. Anderson's time and efforts but feels like a total fool instead. What is he doing here? How can Mr. McGregor believe in me when I am such a loser? thinks Tom.

Seeing Tom's awkwardness, Sam decides to change track. "Tell me what it is you like about your job, Tom?" asks Sam.

"Oh, Mr. Anderson, I like everything about the department store. The store carries the best quality clothing anywhere in town. I like selecting outfits to put on display. That's fun. I like watching how clothes change people," he adds.

"How do clothes change people, Tom?" asks Sam with curiosity.

Laughing, Tom says, "Some women come in and say they need 'retail therapy' and do lots of shopping. As they find outfits that they look great in, their spirits start to lift, and they aren't as sad and depressed as when they came into the store."

"Hum," thinks Sam. "What about men?"

"Men, well, I don't think men do as much retail therapy as women. I think men end up in bars. The men that do shop seem to gravitate to clothing that makes them look sexy and desirable or stylish, successful, and prosperous."

Sam is impressed that Tom is observant and seems to be aware of the customers' motivations for shopping.

"Tom, Mr. McGregor says that you aren't always on time to work."

Tom slides back in his chair, looks down at his hands again, and is embarrassed. What can he say? It's true. He knows enough not to try to justify his lateness. Mr. McGregor says they are just excuses and reasons instead of results.

Finally, Tom says, "I don't know why Mr. McGregor believes in me. I seem to mess up a lot. My mom is right. She tells me all the time that I will never amount to much. I'm trying the best that I can, but I still screw up," says a sad Tom.

"Tell me if I'm right Tom," says Mr. Anderson, with gentleness in his voice. "You feel incompetent, unimportant, and worthless. You feel that you will never be good enough, smart enough, or successful. You don't allow yourself any dreams or goals because they would never come true. Is that about it?"

As Mr. Anderson speaks, Tom can feel his embarrassment increase. His throat closes, and he fights back the tears. He wants to run out of Mr. Anderson's office, but his legs will not support him if he tries to stand.

"Tom, I do a process with my clients called EFT tapping. EFT stands for Emotional Freedom Technique. I would like to teach you how to tap now and do some tapping. Are you game?"

Not able to speak, Tom shakes his head in the affirmative.

Mr. Anderson and Tom tap:
* Even though it's not okay for my life to change, I totally and completely accept myself.
* Even though I feel incompetent, unimportant, and worthless, I totally and completely accept myself
* Even though I will never be good enough, smart enough, or successful, I totally and completely accept myself.
* Even though my dreams and goals will never come true, I totally and completely accept myself.

Tom can feel himself becoming more relaxed after each tapping. He feels himself shifting in his chair, maybe sitting a little taller. He likes the tapping thing. It is better than answering questions that he doesn't have answers for. He isn't quite as sad.

"This week, Tom, I want you to think about this: If you could have anything you wanted, even if it was impossible, what would it be?"

"Are you talking work-related?" asks Tom.

"It can be work-related or not work-related," says Sam. He deliberately leaves it wide open to see if and where Tom's mind wanders.

Back at the store later that morning, Mr. McGregor asks Tom to come to his office before he leaves for the day. All day, Tom wonders what he did wrong that would make him have to stop by Mr. McGregor's office. Had Mr. Anderson mentioned anything to him about not being good enough, smart enough, or feeling incompetent? Mr. Anderson said that he wouldn't be discussing the sessions together with Mr. McGregor. Tom feels on edge all day long. He works extra hard, so Mr. McGregor won't think of him as incompetent.

At the end of the day, Tom raps on Mr. McGregor's office door. "Come in, Tom," answers a cheerful Mr. McGregor.

Good sign, thinks Tom. He's not angry or upset. He actually seems happy. Maybe this won't be so bad. Perhaps, I'm not getting fired.

Robert begins, "Tom, I have been wanting to expand our young adult section of the store, specifically young men of your age. Next week, I'm going on a 3-day buying trip, and I would like you to come with me. We would leave first thing Monday morning and be back Wednesday night. Do you think this is something that you might like to do with me?"

"Me, really?" says an astounded Tom. "Are you sure it's me who you want to go with you? I mean this is something Ricky or Dave could probably do much better than me."

Laughing, Robert says, "Is that a yes, or no?"

Without hesitation, Tom says, "Yes."

Smiling, Robert says, "I was hoping that you would say yes. Go down to Men's Suits and select two different suits, three shirts, and three ties for the trip. Charge the items to the store. Mac is waiting for you to help you with your selection."

Tom's eyes go wide with surprise. Two suits, three shirts, and ties, and charge the store? Did he just win the lottery?

Robert had given Mac, a fine Irish man with a twinkle in his eye and a full head of auburn hair, instructions to "assist Tom," but allow him to make his selections. Robert wants to see what choices Tom will make.

Mac treats Tom like he is royalty, a man of distinction. At first, Tom is embarrassed to be waited on and treated with such respect, until Mac says, "Lad, if you want to be standing next to Mr. McGregor and representing McGregor's Department Store, you need to dress as such. You wouldn't want to be embarrassing him, would you?"

"No!" Tom says. "I don't want him to regret asking me on this trip!"

"Aye," says Mac.

Tom has long admired the fine clothing that McGregor's sells. He does not want to embarrass Mr. McGregor. Tom stands up tall and tells Mac the suits that he wants to try on. While Mac is finding the suits, Tom selects several ties and shirts to try on with the suits. A whole hour later, Mac is ringing up Tom's selection, and Tom signs his name on the sales receipt.

When Tom leaves, Mac calls Robert to report. "He will make you proud, Mr. McGregor. He has fine taste in the selections that he made. Huh!" Chuckling, Mac adds, "Generation Z?

Millennials? Guess calling them young lads is old-fashioned these days."

Early Monday morning, Tom arrives at the store with his suits, ties, and shirts packed at the appointed time. No way was he going to be late for this trip, this opportunity. He is actually early since he hardly slept the night before. Tom doesn't remember being so excited about anything, ever, in his life.

During the whole trip, Tom listens and watches everything that Mr. McGregor does and says. At first, he is afraid to voice his opinion, for fear that he will say the wrong thing. When Mr. McGregor tells Tom that he, Mr. McGregor, will be making the final decisions, but he values Tom's insight into what young men his age are wearing, Tom becomes more relaxed and forthright in giving his honest opinions.

At his next session with Mr. Anderson, excitedly Tom shares, "I can't believe that Mr. McGregor asked me to go along with him on a buying trip for clothes. He wants to expand the clothing selections for the millennials and generation z."

"Wow. What did you think?" asks Sam.

"We ate in fancy restaurants. We rode around in limos with chauffeurs. Everyone was so nice to us." Shaking his head side to side, Tom continues, "I never knew a world like that existed. Yeah, you know, you see it in the movies and on TV, but it was totally different to actually experience it! For real!"

"How did your parents respond when you told them?" asks Mr. Anderson.

"My dad was excited for me." Looking down at his hands, Tom adds, "My mom told me that I would screw it up and embarrass myself." Glancing up at Sam, he says, "Mr. Anderson, I did not screw it up. I watched everything that Mr. McGregor did and tried to do the same things."

Shifting the topic, Sam asks, "Tom, did you think about the homework that I assigned to you last week?"

"The one where I had to think about what I would do or want and it could be absolutely anything?" Again, Tom looks down at his hands, his excitement now gone. "Well, I tried. I have no control over what happens in my life. It's better not to dream. That's what my mom says. If I have dreams, she says that I will only be disappointed. She says that life is tough, then you die."

"Sounds like this might be a good time to tap," Mr. Anderson says, and they tapped.

* Even though I have no control over what happens in my life, I totally and completely accept myself.
* Even though I would only be disappointed if I had dreams, I totally and completely accept myself.
* Even though my dreams will never become a reality, I totally and completely accept myself.
* Even though I am not talented enough to be successful, I totally and completely accept myself.

At the end of the session, Mr. Anderson writes out Tom's homework:

* Even though I am reluctant to set goals, I totally and completely accept myself.

* Even though I have no clue what I want in life, I totally and completely accept myself.
* Even though I am not aware of my options or choices, I totally and completely accept myself.
* Even though my goals never happen, I totally and completely accept myself.
* Even though I am a mistake, I totally and completely accept myself.
* Even though I'm defective and full of flaws, I totally and completely accept myself.

Tom becomes more confident as the weeks progress. Mr. McGregor asks his opinion on how to display the merchandise and how to appeal to the millennial shopper. With Mr. Anderson, he explores how broken, lost, and confused he has felt. He continues to tap with Mr. Anderson and has tapping homework:

* I don't believe in myself.
* I don't go after what I want.
* What I want doesn't matter.
* I am inadequate and broken.
* I am not in charge of my life.
* I don't see myself as a winner.
* I don't live up to my potential.
* I feel lost, confused, and afraid.
* I have difficulty asserting myself.
* I am not smart, talented, or capable.
* I have difficulty asking for what I want.

About three months after starting sessions with Mr. Anderson, Tom begins to have a clear vision of what he wants for himself. Feeling more confident than ever before, Tom knocks on Mr. McGregor's door and asks if he can talk with him.

"Sure Tom. Come in. Let me just finish this email. Have a seat while I do." Once the email is sent, he turns his attention to Tom and asks what's on his mind.

Feeling a little shaky and scared, but acting totally confident, Tom starts, "Mr. McGregor, I want to talk to you about my future here at the store."

Inwardly smiling, Robert says, "I'm all ears. Let's talk about your future here at the store. What might that be?"

"Glad you asked," says Tom. "I have a lot of ideas for the young men's department—fashion shows and other ways to market the department, including social media to bring in the 20-something buyer. I want to do more than just sell or display the merchandise. I want to be a part of the marketing team." Tom takes a deep breath and decides that he will wait for Mr. McGregor to think and maybe comment on what he said.

Leaning back in his chair, Robert studies Tom to see if the confidence is real or a façade. He waits to see if Tom stands his ground and has the courage to pursue his request.

Tom waits as Mr. McGregor thinks about his desire to be a part of the marketing team. He remains silent, waiting to answer any question that Mr. McGregor might have. Tom's intent is clear in his mind about what he wants. With Mr. Anderson's guidance, he is able to feel worthy, valued, and motivated. He is able to breathe life into dreams that had been deflated a long time ago. He feels confidence that he never knew he had. Tom is ready for his life to change in the direction of his choosing.

Finally, Mr. McGregor says, "Okay, Tom, let's see what you can do. Set up a meeting with Harold in the marketing department and present your ideas to him."

With a huge smile on his face, Tom says that he will and floats out of the room.

The following day is his session with Mr. Anderson. "I did it, Mr. Anderson. I talked to Mr. McGregor, and he told me to set up an appointment with Harold, the head of marketing. Three months ago, I felt lost, and now I feel like I have found something that I am passionate about."

"You were willing to do the work, Tom. Mr. McGregor believed in you from the beginning. Now, I know you also believe in yourself," says a happy Sam Anderson.

"Oh," triumphantly, Tom announces, "I am moving out! My best friend from high school called last night. He graduates from college in a few weeks and wants to return home. He wants us to room together."

"Wow. Sounds like our work together has come to an end. What do you think?" says Mr. Anderson.

"Mr. Anderson, I would not be where I am today without your help and EFT tapping. Thank you so much. If I get hung up, can I come back for a session or two on my dime? Not Mr. McGregor's."

"Tom, you are my type of client, one that is willing to explore themselves and do the work necessary to make the changes that they want in their lives. It would be a pleasure to stay in touch and get you 'unhinged' when needed!"

Chapter 3
Discovering EFT Tapping

Our behavior, what we do and say, is determined by our beliefs. Beliefs precede all of our actions, reactions, thoughts, feelings, experiences, and habits.

In 2000, Johnnie was one of my life coaching clients. A life coach is someone who works with their clients to identify their goals, and the steps and tasks needed to accomplish their objectives. As much as Johnnie wanted to perform the steps to accomplish his goals, week after week, he was not able to.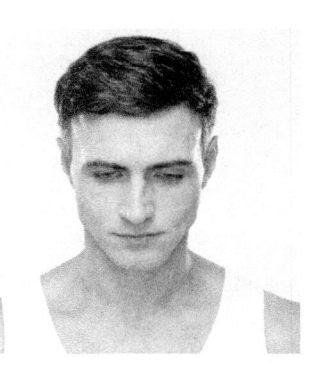

Johnnie's main issue was not feeling good enough about himself. As a result, he withdrew from society, made himself wrong whenever he "messed up," and was a perfectionist.

Johnnie wasn't the only client struggling to fulfill their weekly assignments. I knew underneath the "not feeling good enough" were dysfunctional beliefs and I needed a tool or technique, something, to help my clients move beyond their stumbling blocks.

On a whim, I introduced tapping to Johnnie. I had just finished reading a book on EFT, Emotional Freedom Technique, and was doubtful about its effectiveness. I did not know how tapping one's head would change their life. I did know from what I read that tapping could change dysfunctional beliefs on a subconscious level. I thought, "Nothing ventured, nothing gained."

The following appointment, Johnnie reported back that he had gone to lunch with a group of his fellow employees to celebrate someone's birthday. He had been asked numerous times to accompany them to functions away from the office before, and every time Johnnie declined. He was sure other people saw him as he saw himself, not good enough.

He was amazed. First, that he went to lunch and second, he actually enjoyed himself. He contributed the shift in himself to the tapping. "That's the only thing different between last week and this week," he told me. I was surprised he actually went to lunch, enjoyed himself, and that tapping made a difference.

During that session, Johnnie and I talked about the beliefs that he felt contributed to not feeling good enough and less than others. It was eye-opening for me and shifted the way I conducted sessions.

To change our lives, we need to address the underlying cause of an issue. We need to uncover dysfunctional beliefs, and then, eliminate them from the subconscious.

A belief is accepting something to be true, whether it is Truth or not. A dysfunctional belief is a belief that takes us away from peace, love, joy, stability, acceptance, and harmony. It causes us to feel stressed, fearful, anxious, and/or insecure.

Beliefs are "stored" in the subconscious mind. The subconscious is the part of the mind responsible for all of our involuntary actions, like our heartbeat and breathing rate. It does not evaluate, make decisions, or pass judgment. It just is. It does not determine if something is "right" or "wrong."

The subconscious is much like the software of a computer. Just as a computer can only do what it has been programmed to do, we can only do as we are programmed to do.

Our programming is determined by our beliefs. Beliefs and memories are "stored" in the subconscious.

The conscious mind is the part of us that thinks, passes judgments, makes decisions, remembers, analyzes, has desires, and communicates with others. It is responsible for logic and reasoning, understanding and comprehension. The mind determines our actions, feelings, thoughts, judgments, and decisions based on our beliefs.

EFT TAPPING

EFT Tapping, Emotional Freedom Technique, is a tool that allows us to change dysfunctional beliefs and emotions on a subconscious level. It involves making a statement while tapping different points along traditional Chinese meridian pathways.

The general principle behind EFT is that the cause of all negative emotions is a disruption in the body's energy system. By tapping on locations where several different meridians flow, we can release unproductive memories, emotions, and beliefs that cause the blockages.

After the shift in Johnnie and other clients, I was determined to discover how to utilize EFT Tapping to help other clients effectively eliminate dysfunctional beliefs. After teaching tapping to ten clients, I had all the clients come in for a group session. We called it Discovery Evening and spent a fun evening exploring different aspects of tapping to determine how to maximize results. My livelihood was dependent on the success of my clients and thus, I was motivated to learn the most effective methods.

This book is the result of twenty-plus years of doing private sessions as well as teaching classes on EFT Tapping and training others to be practitioners.

Chapter 4
Meridian Tapping

EFT is sometimes referred to as meridian tapping or energy tapping.

The circulatory system moves blood throughout the body. The nervous system is a vast network of nerves that sends electrical signals throughout the body. And the respiratory system brings air into and out of the lungs. But what about energy? What system is responsible for generating and moving energy in the body? The circulatory system has arteries and veins, the nervous system has nerves, and the respiratory system uses blood to supply air to the cells of the body. But, what about energy?

In Chinese philosophy, energy is called "chi," (also known as qi, prana, and life force in other cultures). Chi flows through our bodies and is impacted by every thought we think, every word we speak, every action we take, and every belief we hold.

Traditional Chinese Medicine, thousands of years ago, mapped out the energy pathways in the physical body. These pathways called meridians. Meridians are pathways in which energy travels throughout the body. Think super highway! Think rivers and streams.

When blood and oxygen are able to flow unobstructed, the body is healthy. If there are any restrictions to blood or oxygen flow, illness will result. When an accident happens on a super highway, the flow of traffic is impacted. When rivers and streams become polluted with debris, water stops flowing.

When energy is able to flow freely, unobstructed, the body is healthy. Dis-ease happens when the energy is blocked. Every breath, emotion, and thought reflects the state and quality of our chi. Energy can become blocked by our thoughts, speech, actions, and beliefs as well as stress, injury, and trauma.

Tapping on different points along the energy pathways has the potential to release blocked energy. This is the principle behind EFT Tapping. EFT Tapping activates points along the meridian pathways to release blockages so that energy flows more freely and health is restored.

Chapter 5
How to Tap

There is a long form and a short form of tapping. At our Discovery Evening, we tapped both forms to determine if one was more successful than the other. There was no difference. Both were effective regardless of the dysfunctional belief or emotion we were exploring. Below are the instructions for tapping the short form of EFT Tapping.

EFT Tapping involves 1) making a statement and 2) tapping.

THE EFT TAPPING STATEMENT WE SAY AS WE TAP

An EFT Tapping Statement has three parts:

Part 1: starts with **"Even though"** followed by

Part 2: a statement which could be the **dysfunctional emotion or belief**, and

Part 3: ends with **"I totally and completely accept myself."**

A complete statement would be, **"Even though I fear change, I totally and completely accept myself."**

TAPPING INSTRUCTIONS

There are two different segments of the tapping. The first is called "the setup," and the second is the tapping. The following instructions are for the right hand. Reverse the directions to tap using the left hand. It is more effective, to tap only one side rather than both sides simultaneously.

I. Setup

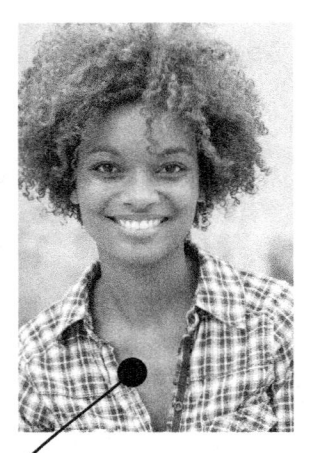

A. With the fingertips of the right hand, find a tender spot below the left collarbone. Once the tender spot is identified, press firmly on the spot, moving the fingertips in a clockwise, circular motion.

Tender spot below the left collarbone

B. As the fingers circle and press against the tender spot, repeat the tapping statement three times: "Even though, [tapping statement]___, I totally and completely accept myself."

An example would be: "Even though I fear change, I totally and completely accept myself."

II. TAPPING

A. After repeating the statement three times, tap the following eight points, repeating the [tapping statement] at each point. Tap each point five – ten times:

1. The inner edge of the eyebrow, just above the eye. [I fear change.]
2. Temple, just to the side of the eye. [I fear change.]
3. Just below the eye (on the cheekbone). [I fear change.]
4. Under the nose. [I fear change.]
5. Under the lips. [I fear change.]
6. Under the knob of the collar bone. [I fear change.]
7. Three inches under the arm pit. [I fear change.]
8. Top back of the head. [I fear change.]

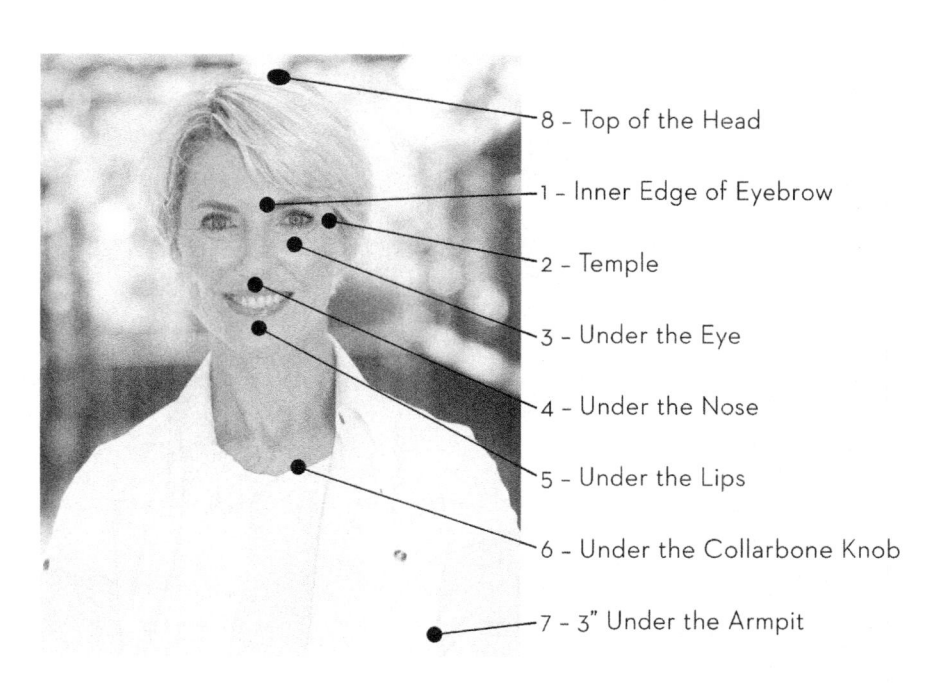

8 – Top of the Head

1 – Inner Edge of Eyebrow

2 – Temple

3 – Under the Eye

4 – Under the Nose

5 – Under the Lips

6 – Under the Collarbone Knob

7 – 3" Under the Armpit

B. After tapping, take a deep breath. If you are not able to take a deep, full, satisfying breath, do eye rolls.

III. Eye Rolls

A. With one hand, tap continuously on the back of the other hand between the fourth and fifth fingers.
B. Hold your head straight forward, eyes looking straight down.
C. For six seconds, roll your eyes from the floor straight up toward the ceiling while repeating the tapping statement. Keep your head straight forward, only moving your eyes.

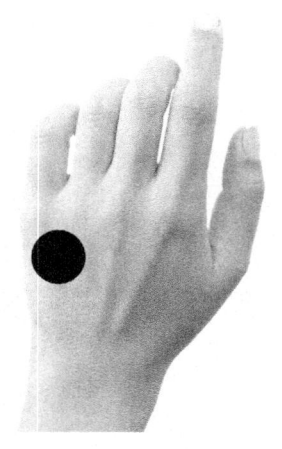

IV. take a deep breath

A. If you are able to take a deep breath or if you yawn, the statement cleared.
B. If you are not able to take a deep breath, there might be other dysfunctional beliefs or emotions that need to be addressed as well.

ALTERNATIVE TO TAPPING

An alternative to tapping the eight points is to tap the side of the hand, also known as the karate chop point.

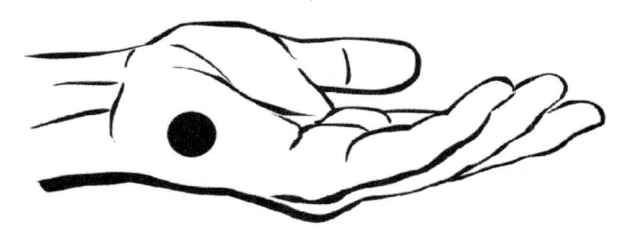

I TOTALLY AND COMPLETELY ACCEPT MYSELF OR
I TOTALLY AND COMPLETELY LOVE AND ACCEPT MYSELF.

At the end of the tapping statement, we say: "I totally and completely accept myself." Some practitioners include "love myself." What the Discovery group learned is not everyone loves themselves, and it was difficult for some to make the statement. They paused and cringed every time they said, "I totally and completely love myself."

One client said, "I just can't say that because I know it isn't true. Every time I say, 'I love myself,' I am reminded that I don't and then feel guilty that I don't, and maybe the tapping won't work because I am lying to myself. I can accept myself, but in terms of loving myself, I'm not there yet."

I took notice when others said they felt the same way. For tapping to be most effective, it was best for some to say, "I totally and completely accept myself," rather than, "I totally and completely love and accept myself." The majority of the Discovery

Evening group preferred to leave love out of the statement, so the statement they said was, "I totally and completely accept myself."

The last part of the statement, whether that is "I totally and completely accept myself" or "I totally and completely love and accept myself," is a matter of preference by the tapper.

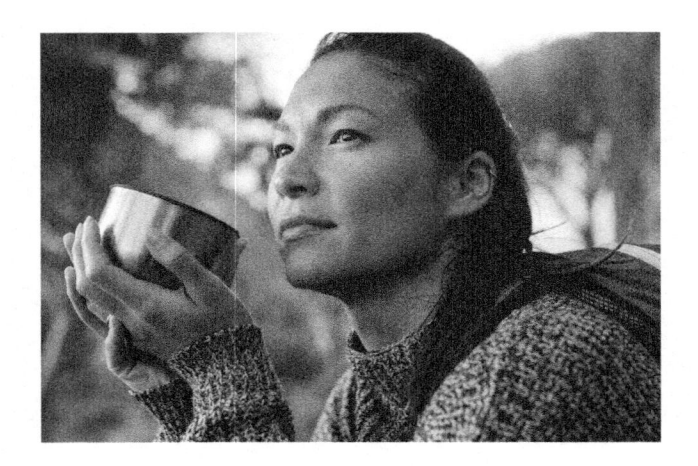

Chapter 6
What We Say as We Tap Is VERY Important!

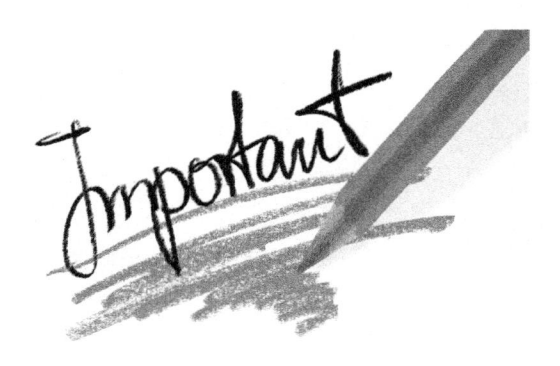

Before the explanation of how and why tapping works, there are several other aspects of tapping that I would like to discuss. One aspect is the tapping statement.

During our Discovery Evening, we experimented with different tapping statements and were able to determine which tapping statements were most effective.

All of our beliefs are programmed into our subconscious minds. If we want to change our lives, we must delete dysfunctional beliefs and emotions on a subconscious level. The statements we say as we tap are the instructions for the subconscious mind and need to be stated in such a way that the unhealthy belief or emotions will be eliminated.

The tapping statements we say as we tap are critical

Example: You get in a taxi. Several hours later, you still have not arrived at your destination. "*Why?*" you ask. Because you did not give the destination to the taxi driver!

Tapping without an adequate tapping statement is like riding in a cab without giving the cab driver our destination!

TWO CRITICAL ASPECTS OF THE TAPPING STATEMENT

1. TAPPING STATEMENTS THAT AGREE WITH THE CURRENT DYSFUNCTIONAL BELIEF ARE MOST EFFECTIVE.

If the statement we verbalize as we tap does not agree with the current dysfunctional belief, we could end up sabotaging the tapping by forgetting the statement or with other distractions.

For example, you don't feel empowered. You feel like a coward, a failure, and a wimp. If the tapping statement is "I am empowered," the body will remind you that you aren't powerful and not only are you not powerful, but you are also a coward, a failure, and a wimp. If, instead, we tap, "I am not powerful," this statement agrees with the current dysfunctional belief.

The body is less likely to sabotage an EFT Tapping statement that agrees with the current belief.

During the Discovery Evening, as one client was tapping, he stopped in the middle of tapping and said, "It's raining outside." It had been raining all day. It didn't just start raining. This tapper was totally distracted by the rain. The group chuckled, and a discussion followed. We realized the tapping statement needed to agree with the current dysfunctional belief, memory, or emotion to be effective.

The body is here to protect us based on our beliefs, functional or dysfunctional. If the current belief is "I am not powerful," if we were to tap, "I am powerful," the body knows this to not be true and thus, could distract us or sabotage the tapping in some way. The body is less likely to sabotage the tapping and the process if the EFT Tapping statement agrees with the current belief.

2. SUBCONSCIOUS MIND AND TAPPING STATEMENTS

The middle section of the tapping statements are instructions for the subconscious mind. When tapping, we only care what the subconscious hears. There are three rules of the subconscious mind that I like. "The three P Rules."

THREE RULES OF THE SUBCONSCIOUS MIND

1. Personal. It only understands "I," "me," "myself." First-person.

2. Positive. The subconscious does not hear the word "no." When you say, "I am not going to eat that piece of cake," the subconscious hears, "Yummm! Cake! I am going to eat a piece of that cake!"

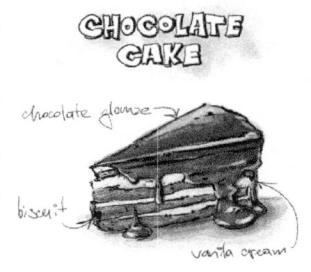

3. Present time. Time does not exist for the subconscious. The only time it knows is "now," present time. "I'm going to clean the garage tomorrow." Tomorrow never comes thus, we constantly put off cleaning the garage.

We tried different types of tapping statements at the Discovery Evening. As my clients were tapping, "I am powerful," many of them found their minds wandering and distracted so much so they forgot what they were tapping.

When we added the word "not" to the tapping statement, "I am not powerful," there were a lot of yawns. A yawn is a signal from the body that a tapping statement cleared. We continued with more statements and added a "no" or "not" to the statement and had tremendous results.

When the statement is "I am not powerful," the "**not**" appeases the physical body, and the subconscious hears, "I am powerful!" Now, my clients only want to tap statements that include a "no" or "not" in the statements. They think tapping statements with a "no" or "not" are brilliant. I agree.

As tappers, we only care what the subconscious hears. It does not hear the word "no."

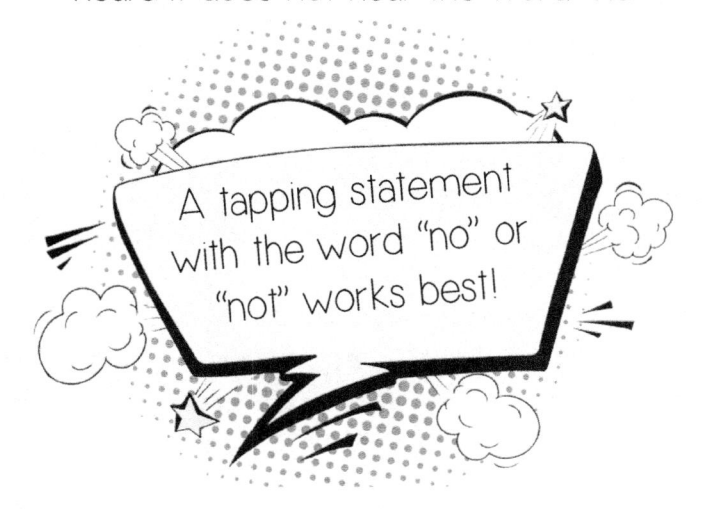

A tapping statement with the word "no" or "not" works best!

Chapter 7
Pattern Interrupt

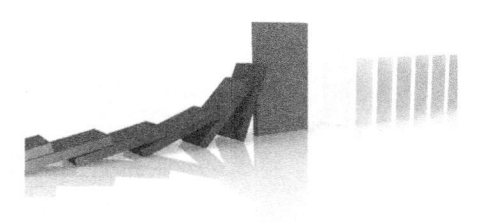

Another topic I want to discuss before moving on to how and why EFT Tapping works is "pattern interrupt." A pattern interrupt is an NLP, neuro-linguistic programming, term. It is anything that creates an abrupt change.

You are having a conversation with a friend. Mid-sentence, they stop talking, reach out and put their hand on your arm. You are startled when the conversation comes to an abrupt end. Even more surprised when they put their hand on your arm. Pattern interrupt.

Part of the effectiveness of tapping is the "pattern interrupt" of energy flowing along the meridians. Dysfunctional beliefs, painful memories, and past traumas can block energy from flowing freely. Tapping on various energy points can release stagnant and blocked energy. When energy is able to flow freely, health is restored. When healthy, the body will automatically gravitate to well-being, prosperity, and happiness. In a confused state, it is difficult to know our Truths, the nitty-gritty of ourselves. By tapping, we become more of who we are and who we are meant to be as the blocks are released.

This might be a good time to also discuss tapping on one side or both sides simultaneously. In traditional Chinese medicine, there are twelve major meridians that run on each side of the body, one side mirroring the other.

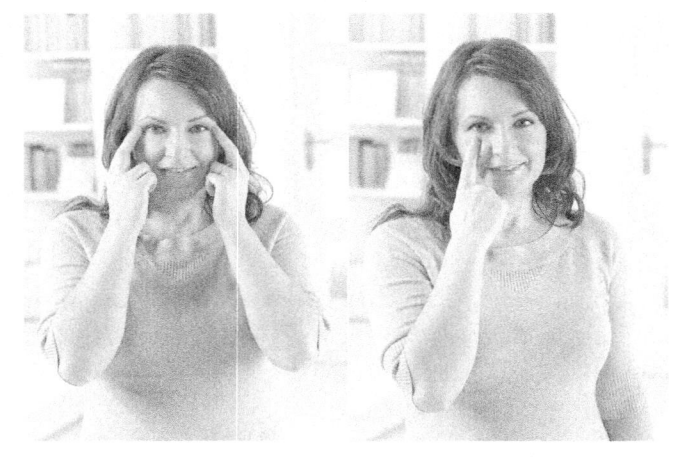

Most Effective

When the Discovery Evening group tapped both sides simultaneously, most found statements were not clearing. However, when they only tapped one side at a time, statements were clearing and there were a lot of yawns. The group and I concluded that tapping one side was more effective than tapping both sides. Tapping both sides was not as much of a pattern interrupt since the meridians flow on both sides. Tapping one side was more of a pattern interrupt.

Chapter 8
How Does EFT Tapping Work?

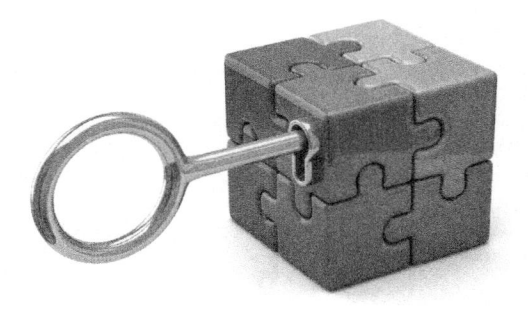

Having an understanding of an EFT Tapping statement and a pattern interrupt might help you comprehend how EFT Tapping actually works.

1. ACCEPTANCE: The last part of the tapping statement, we say, "I totally and completely accept myself." Acceptance brings us into present time. We can only heal if we are in present time.

2. ADDRESSES THE CURRENT DYSFUNCTIONAL BELIEFS ON A SUB-CONSCIOUS LEVEL: To make changes in our lives, we have to eliminate dysfunctional beliefs on a subconscious level. The middle part of the tapping statements are the "instructions" for the subconscious.

3. PATTERN INTERRUPT: Dysfunctional memories and/or beliefs block energy from flowing freely along traditional Chinese meridians. Tapping is a pattern interrupt that disrupts the flow of energy to allow our body's own Infinite Wisdom to come forth for healing. For the EFT Tapping statement "I fear change" and the client does fear change:

* This statement agrees with the current dysfunctional belief and, thus appeases the physical body. We won't be distracted as we tap.

* The tapping disrupts the energy flow so our Truth can come forth.

Chapter 9
Benefits of EFT Tapping

EFT Tapping is an evidence-based self-help tool to improve our physical, mental, and emotional well-being. There are over one hundred studies conducted in ten different countries by more than sixty researchers demonstrating EFT Tapping's effectiveness and success.

It can help reduce anxiety, stress, and food cravings. It has proven helpful for those enduring PTSD, depression, addictions, and chronic pain. Tapping can increase energy levels and reduce fatigue. Research has found that it significantly increases athletic performance. It can reduce muscular tension and joint pain. Sleeping better and less pain resulted in greater happiness and joy!

EFT Tapping can change:

Beliefs

Emotions

Self-images

Our story

Thoughts

Mind chatter

Painful memories

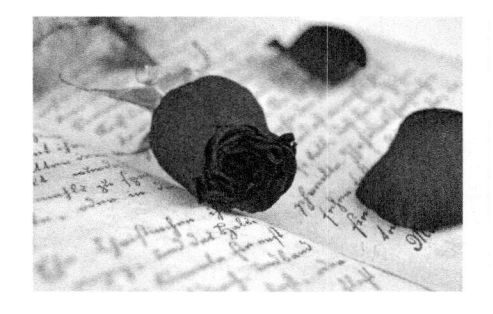

Here Are Ten Benefits of EFT Tapping:

1. Eliminate Dysfunctional Beliefs and Emotions

To transform our lives, we need to delete and/or modify our beliefs on a subconscious level. EFT Tapping has the potential to change our lives by eliminating the unhealthy beliefs and emotions on a subconscious level.

The natural state for the body is health and well-being. Blocked energy causes dis-ease. When we cut our finger, our body knows how to heal the cut itself. Once dysfunctional emotions, experiences, and beliefs have been "deleted," our body automatically gravitates to health, wealth, peace, love, and joy.

2. Reduce Stress and Anxiety

Research has shown that tapping can significantly decrease cortisol (stress hormone) levels and quiet the amygdala (stress center in the brain). This helps us to feel calmer and think more clearly. Less stress led to improved sleep which resulted in feeling more energized and less fatigued. The resting heart 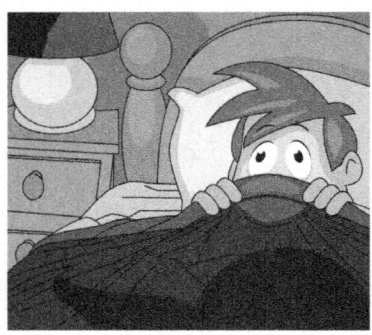 rate and blood pressure were reduced as well.

3. Changes Are Permanent

Once an unhealthy, dysfunctional belief has been eliminated, the body automatically gravitates to well-being. As a result, the changes we make with EFT are permanent.

4. Diminish Food Cravings and Increase Weight Loss

A study of ninety-six overweight adults was conducted in 2018. After four weeks of tapping, brain scans showed changes in the part of the brain associated with cravings. The participants reported less interest in food. Tapping can help with weight loss by creating changes in parts of the brain that activate food cravings.

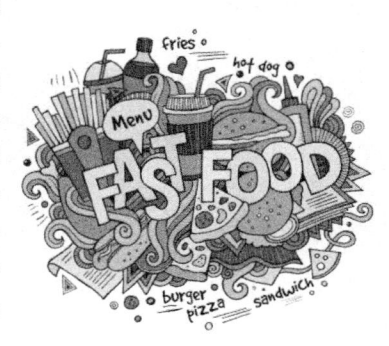

Overeating and emotional eating are symptoms of unresolved issues underneath the desire to eat. Not only has tapping been found to help cope with the physical urge to binge and emotionally eat, but it has also helped to heal the core issues around the need to overeat.

5. Improved Emotional Well-being
By eliminating the unhealthy beliefs that result in anger, fear, and/or sadness, we feel happier, our attitudes improve, and we are more optimistic about life.

6. Post Traumatic Stress Disorder (PTSD) and Other Traumas

PTSD is not limited to war veterans. Involvement in any sort of accident, surviving a natural disaster, school shootings, being told one has a terminal disease, victims of assault including sexual assault, all of these can leave one traumatized and suffering from PTSD.

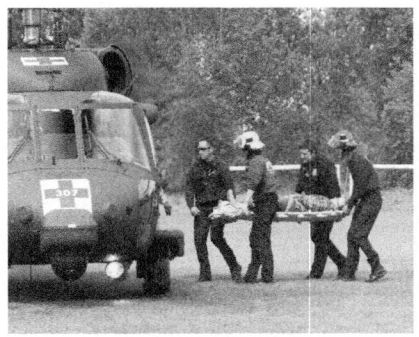 PTSD has been the subject of many studies. Research studies have found that EFT Tapping significantly decreased and/or resolved participants' PTSD, reducing flashbacks and nightmares, insomnia, trouble concentrating, isolation, hypervigilance, and aggression.

In a 2013 study, 60% of war vets felt their PTSD had been resolved after three tapping sessions. Another 30% felt their PTSD had been resolved after six tapping sessions.

7. Desensitize Emotions

We might have a difficult person in our life that ignores and/or criticizes us, so we tap the statement: "This difficult person [or their name] ignores and criticizes me."

Tapping does not mean they will no longer ignore and/or criticize us; however, it can desensitize us, so we are no longer affected by their behavior. Once we have desensitized the emotions, our perception and mental thinking improves. We are better able to make informed decisions. We don't take and make everything personal. Our health is not negatively impacted. Our hearts no longer beat 100 beats/minute, smoke stops coming out of our ears, and our faces don't turn red with anger and frustration anymore.

8. Reduce Pain and Headaches

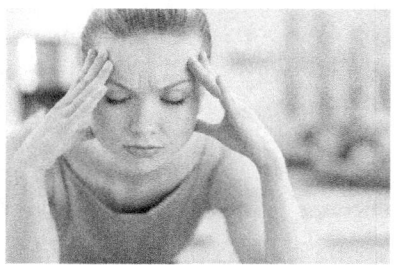

Numerous research studies have found that EFT Tapping has helped to reduce the frequency and severity of headaches as well as reduce chronic pain.

One study of people suffering from frequent tension-type headaches found that routine tapping twice a day for two months reduced both the frequency and intensity of tension headaches.

In another study of people with fibromyalgia, participants found that after an eight-week tapping program, their levels of pain were reduced.

Another study focused on people who had just undergone surgery. Five minutes of tapping for three days post-surgery significantly decreased pain levels compared to those who received no tapping treatment.

9. Athletic Performance

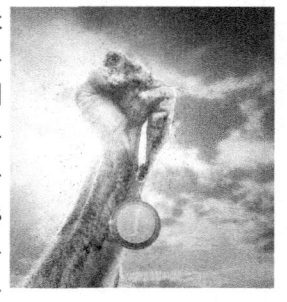

Various research studies have found that EFT Tapping has improved athletic performance. One study with female and male basketball players showed improved performance after fifteen minutes of EFT Tapping compared to players who did not tap. Another study with soccer players showed significant improvement in goal scoring as a result of tapping. With other athletes, EFT Tapping helped their mental mindset, increased self-confidence, and reduced performance anxiety.

10. Boost the Immune System
EFT Tapping has been shown to increase the production of white blood cells which can supercharge our immune system.

As an EFT Practitioner, I have used EFT Tapping to help clients experience all of the benefits listed here and have witnessed the remarkable improvement in their lives. My clients have benefited from tapping for issues that include weight loss, emotional eating, athletic performance, chronic pain, and PTSD as well as personal empowerment issues.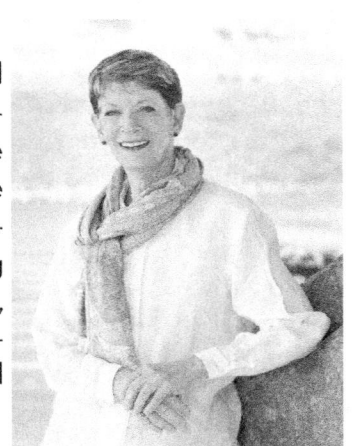

Chapter 10
The Very First EFT Tapping
Statement to Tap

The very first EFT Tapping statement I have clients and students tap is, "It is not okay or safe for my life to change." At the first session with a client, I muscle-test (a technique to ask the body questions bypassing the conscious mind), if it is okay and safe for their lives to change. No one person tested strong, that it was okay or safe for their lives to change.

I have muscle-tested this statement with more than a thousand people. Not one person tested strong that it was okay or safe for their life to change.

How effective can EFT or any therapy be
if it is not okay or safe for our lives to change?

Since our lives are constantly changing, if it is not okay or safe for our lives to change, it creates stress for the body every time it does. Stress creates another whole set of issues for ourselves, our lives, and our bodies.

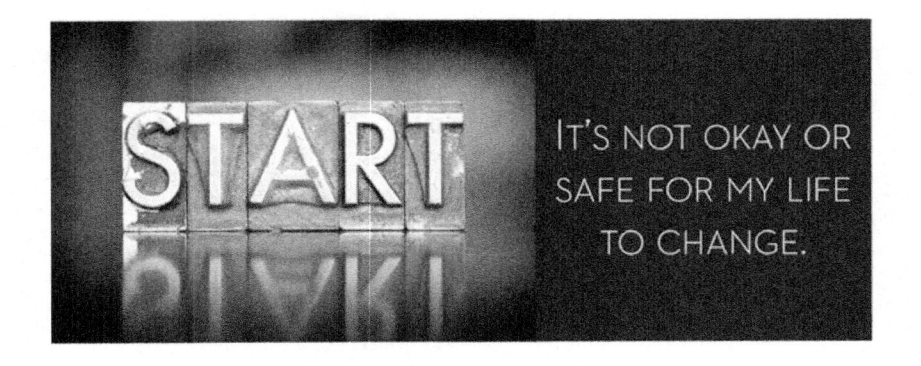

IT'S NOT OKAY OR SAFE FOR MY LIFE TO CHANGE.

Chapter 11
Yawning and Taking a Deep Breath

From traditional Chinese Medicine, we know that when chi (energy) flows freely through the meridians, the body is healthy and balanced. When the energy is blocked, it can result in physical, mental, and/or emotional illness.

Dysfunctional beliefs and emotions block energy from flowing freely in the body.

With EFT Tapping, as we tap, we release the blocks. As blocked energy is able to flow more freely, the body can now "breathe a sigh of relief." Yawning is that sigh of relief.

If, after tapping, we can take a complete, deep, full, and satisfying breath, we know that an EFT Tapping statement has cleared.

If the yawn or breath is not a full, deep breath then the statement did not clear completely.

Chapter 12
Integration...What Happens After Tapping

After tapping, our system needs some downtime for integration to take place. When the physical body and the mind are "idle," integration can take place.

Sometimes, in the first 24 hours after tapping, we might find ourselves sleeping more than normal or feeling more tired. This downtime is needed to integrate the new changes.

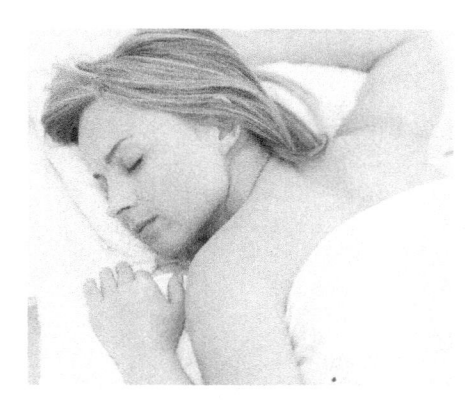

After installing a new program on our computer, sometimes we have to reboot the computer (shut down and restart) for the new program to be integrated into the system.

After tapping, our bodies need to reboot. We need some downtime. When we sleep, the new changes are integrated.

HEALING BEGINS NATURALLY AFTER THE BODY
HAS HAD A CHANCE TO INTEGRATE.

Sometimes, after tapping, we forget the intensity of our pain and think that feeling better has nothing to do with tapping. Something so simple could not possibly be the reason for the improvement!

When we cut our finger, once it is healed, we don't remember cutting our finger. As we move toward health, wealth, and well-being, sometimes we don't remember how unhappy, restless, or isolated we once felt.

I had a client, Sam. He had been struggling with an issue for twenty years. After the session, I called Sam to make sure he was okay. He said, "I'm doing great. I don't know why I needed to see you because I am all good now."

A little confused, I asked if something had happened or what he felt had caused the change to make everything great now. He said, "No." He couldn't imagine that tapping his head would change an issue he had been struggling with for twenty years!

Tapping is a simple exercise that has long-lasting,
meaningful results for a tapper

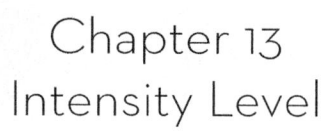

Chapter 13
Intensity Level

One measure of knowing how much an issue has improved is by giving the issue an intensity number (IL) between 1 and 10, 1 being low and with 10 being high. This is done before tapping begins and reassessed throughout the tapping process.

For example, we want a romantic partnership, yet we haven't met "the one." Thinking about a romantic relationship happening, what is the likelihood, on a scale of 1 – 10, with 10 being very likely and 1, not likely at all, of a romantic relationship happening.

After thinking about it, and checking with our inner self, we give ourselves a 2 for the likelihood of a romantic relationship happening. Now, let's start tapping.

When asked what the issues might be, "Well," we say, "It does not seem as if the people I want, want me."

Great tapping statement. Tap, "Even though the people I want don't want me, I totally and completely accept myself." After tapping, we check in with ourselves; the IL has gone up to a 4, so it is now a little bit more likely.

What comes to mind now? "No one will find me desirable." Great tapping statement. "Even though no one will find me desirable, I totally and completely accept myself." Check the IL. How likely? 5. Cool! Progress.

What comes to mind now? "I'm not comfortable being vulnerable in romantic relationships." Great tapping statement. "Even though I'm not comfortable being vulnerable in a romantic relationship, I totally and completely accept myself." Check the IL. Now it is a 6. Still progress.

What comes to mind now? "Well, it feels like if I am in a relationship, I will lose a lot of my freedom." Make this into a tapping statement. "Even though I will lose my freedom when I am in a relationship, I totally and completely accept myself." The IL has gone up to a 7.

What comes to mind now? "Oh, if I was in a relationship, I would have to be accountable to someone!" Make this into a tapping statement: "Even though, I would have to be accountable to someone if I was in a relationship, I totally and completely accept myself." Wow...the IL is 9, very likely!

Chapter 14
Walking Backwards EFT (Backing Up)

As I was working with a client, Joanne, an issue was not clearing. Knowing that movement helps to resolve problems, I told Joanne to stand up. Joanne and I backed up, walking backward, as we spoke the tapping statements. Literally, we walked backwards, step after step, facing forward while our feet stepped backward.

Surprise, surprise, it worked. Every Statement cleared as Joanne backed up.

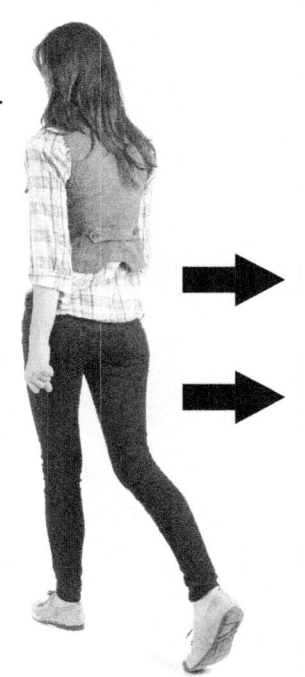

Walking forward represents forward movement in our lives. Walking backward represents the past.

Physical movement can help clear emotional issues and facilitate change.

Walking backward undoes the past and helps to clear, heal, and transform an issue in our lives.

The next client, Bill, came in for his session. I had him walk backwards. His issues were being resolved as well by backing up. Both Joanne and Bill are somewhat athletic and workout. I wanted to know if the backing up would work with non-athletic people. I was teaching an EFT class that night. At the end of the class, we all backed up together. And, IT WORKED!

Let's say we want to process, "I will never be comfortable in the world." Stand up. Make sure nothing is behind you. Then walk backward while facing forward and say, "I will never be comfortable in the world. I will never be comfortable in the world. I will never be comfortable in the world. I will never be comfortable in the world." Repeat the phrase six to eight times.

Initially, as Bill and Joanne began walking backwards, it was difficult for them to keep their balance. As the statement cleared, their balance and ability to walk backwards improved. Joanne exclaimed, "I can tell when the statement begins to clear because I stand taller and my balance improves."

Backing up EFT worked with every client
and student. How cool is that!

Chapter 15
Two Styles of Tapping

Laser-focused Tapping vs Round Robin Tapping

The Discovery Evening group and I explored different issues, situations, and memories to determine how best to resolve and heal different issues in our lives.

With Johnnie not feeling good enough, his situation was more about the beliefs he had about himself. Beliefs such as:

* I will always be rejected because I am not good enough.
* I have to be perfect so others won't see my flaws.
* It's not safe to show others the real me.
* I will never succeed in life.

Kala's situation was different. She had been dating a man for two years and thought he was "the one." She and Steve had talked about marriage, buying a home together, and having a family. They knew each other's likes and dislikes, how they each felt about disciplining children, and what each other's life-long goals were. Kala began reading wedding magazines, and visualizing her wedding gown, and the ceremony.

Three days passed and she had not heard from Steve. She decided to stop by his home. Out front was a "For Rent" sign! A few days later, she received an email from Steve.

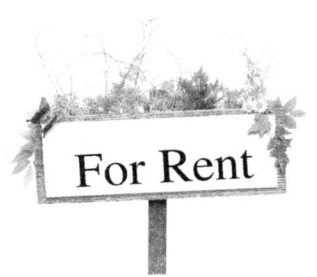

Steve's work offered him a promotion outside the country. He wasn't sure what he wanted to do and didn't want anyone pressuring him to make a decision. He needed to determine what was best for him. Ultimately, he took the new position and ended the relationship with Kala.

Two different situations, each benefitted from a different style of tapping. What the group and I concluded was that "laser-focused tapping," making the same statement for all eight points was best for healing dysfunctional beliefs. The beliefs Johnnie had about "not being good enough" would benefit from this style of tapping.

Round robin tapping, scripts, was best for healing emotions, desensitizing a story, situation, and/or memory. Kala would benefit from the round robin/script tapping to desensitize her crushed heart.

LASER FOCUSED TAPPING
SAME STATEMENT FOR ALL THE TAPPING POINTS IN ONE ROUND

Example: After tapping the statement, "It's not okay for my life to change," if we are able to take a deep breath, we know the statement has cleared. Then if we tap, "I'm not ready for my life to change," and we are not able to take a deep breath, most likely, the statement did not clear.

Circling under the collar bone:

1. Even though, it is not ready for my life to change, I totally and completely accept myself.

2. Even though, it is not ready for my life to change, I totally and completely accept myself.

3. Even though, it is not ready for my life to change, I totally and completely accept myself.

Tapping:

Eyebrow – It's not ready for my life to change.
Temple – It's not ready for my life to change.
Side of the eye - It's not ready for my life to change.
Under the eye – It's not ready for my life to change.
Under the nose – It's not ready for my life to change.
Under the lips – It's not ready for my life to change.
Collar bone knob – It's not ready for my life to change.
Top back of head – It's not ready for my life to change.

Knowing the statement did not clear, we can focus on the reasons, excuses, and/or beliefs about not being ready to change our lives.

* Maybe the changes we need to make would require more of us than we want to give.
* Maybe we don't feel we have the abilities we would need if our life changed.
* Maybe we don't feel our support system, the people in our life, would approve of the changes we want to make.

Follow-up tapping statements for "I'm not ready for my life to change" could be:

* I do not have the abilities change would require.
* I am afraid of change.
* Others will not support the changes I want to make in my life.
* I am not able to make the changes I want to make.
* I do not have the courage that change would require.
* I am too old to change.

Tapping the same statement at all eight points is most effective for clearing beliefs. When a statement does not clear, we can then focus on the reasons, excuses, and/or dysfunctional beliefs that blocked the statement from clearing.

Tapping multiple statements in one round, also known as Scripts or Round Robin tapping, is excellent for healing a story or desensitizing a memory.

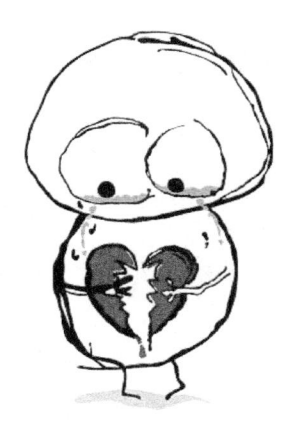

To desensitize the heartache of the break up, the following script/statements could be said, one statement per tapping point:

Eyebrow – My boyfriend broke up with me.

Temple – I am heartbroken.

Side of the eye - He said he doesn't love me anymore.

Under the eye – I don't know how I can go on without him.

Under the nose – It hurts.

Under the lips – I am sad he doesn't love me anymore.

Collar bone knob – I am sad our relationship is over.

Top back of head – I will never find anyone like him ever again.

REFRAMING

Reframing is a Neuro-Linguistic Programming (NLP) term. It is a way to view and experience emotions, situations, and/or behaviors in a more positive manner.

At the end of round robin tapping, we can introduce statements to "reframe" the situation.

An example of reframing could be:

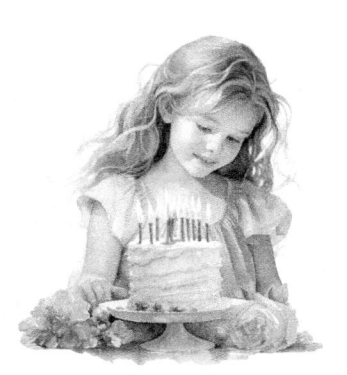

* I want to eat this chocolate cake.
* Maybe eating chocolate is a way to reconnect to my childhood.
* Maybe eating sugar is a way of being loved.
* Maybe I can find a different way of being loved.

Round robin tapping, scripts, can desensitize the hurt and pain. It can heal the pain of our story. It may not rewrite the beliefs. To clear the beliefs, it would be necessary to look at the reasons the relationship didn't work and why our heart is broken or why we crave chocolate.

Round robin/script tapping can also be done by just tapping the side of the hand.

SIDE OF HAND (SOH) TAPPING TO DESENSITIZE A STORY, SITUATION, AND/OR MEMORY

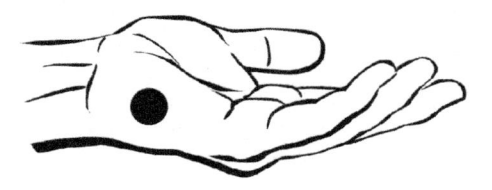

When our lives have been turned upside down and inside out because of something that happened, it is best to neutralize the event. If a memory still haunts us, we can tap the side of the hand as we reflect on the event.

As Sasha, another client of mine, was telling her story, tears filled her eyes. I had her tap the side of her hand as she recalled her worst high school dance ever!

As Sasha tapped the side of the hand, she said: My best friend, Samantha and I, were so excited about attending our first high school dance. We weren't old enough to drive so Sam's dad dropped us off in front of the high school auditorium where the dance was held.

(Continuing to tap the SOH) We were in awe of how the auditorium was transformed into a palace. Sofas were placed around a hardwood dance floor in the center of the room. We promised to be there for each other throughout the night so neither of us would be stranded alone.

(Continuing to tap the SOH) Well, along came Billy McDaniels. Sam had had a crush on Billy since third grade. He asked her to dance. I never saw her again for the rest of the night.

(Continuing to tap the SOH) Those three hours were probably the worst night of my entire life! No one asked me to dance. Every time I joined a group of girls, a new song would begin, and every one of them was asked to dance, everyone except me. I don't know why no one asked me to dance. I felt ugly, abandoned, and undesirable! Talk about being a wallflower. I thought I was invisible. I wanted to hide from embarrassment.

(Continuing to tap the SOH) This was back in the days before cell phones. The auditorium didn't have a payphone to call my parents to come and get me. I had to endure three hours of humiliation, watching every single girl be asked to dance EXCEPT me.

(Continuing to tap the SOH) I never attended another high school dance again!

Whether we tap the side of our hand or the eight tapping points, the result is the same. Round robin tapping can desensitize emotions and memories very effectively.

There are different styles of EFT Tapping.
Find the style that works best for your desired result.

Chapter 16
EFT Tapping Doesn't Work for Me

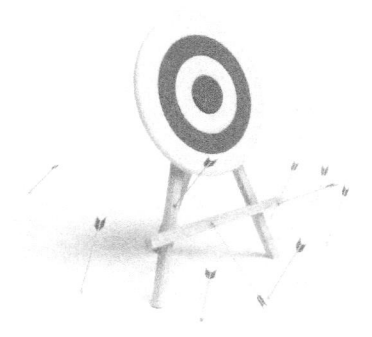

EFT Tapping works best when

1) the statements are worded to eliminate dysfunctional beliefs,
2) the most effective style of tapping is utilized, and
3) we are healing the cause, not just the symptoms.

If an issue doesn't seem to be resolved after tapping, ask yourself the following questions:

* Were the statements worded so that a dysfunctional belief and/or emotion could be addressed and eliminated?

* Was the best style of tapping (laser-focused vs scripts) utilized?

* Were the tapping statements addressing the symptom or the cause?

For EFT Tapping to be effective,
the cause of the issue needs to be healed.

* Having an awareness of our issues does not heal dysfunctional beliefs.
* Forgiving ourselves and/or someone else does not heal dysfunctional beliefs.
* Talk therapy does not heal dysfunctional beliefs.
* Desensitizing emotions does not heal dysfunctional beliefs.
* Healing the experience of a hurtful event does not change dysfunctional beliefs.

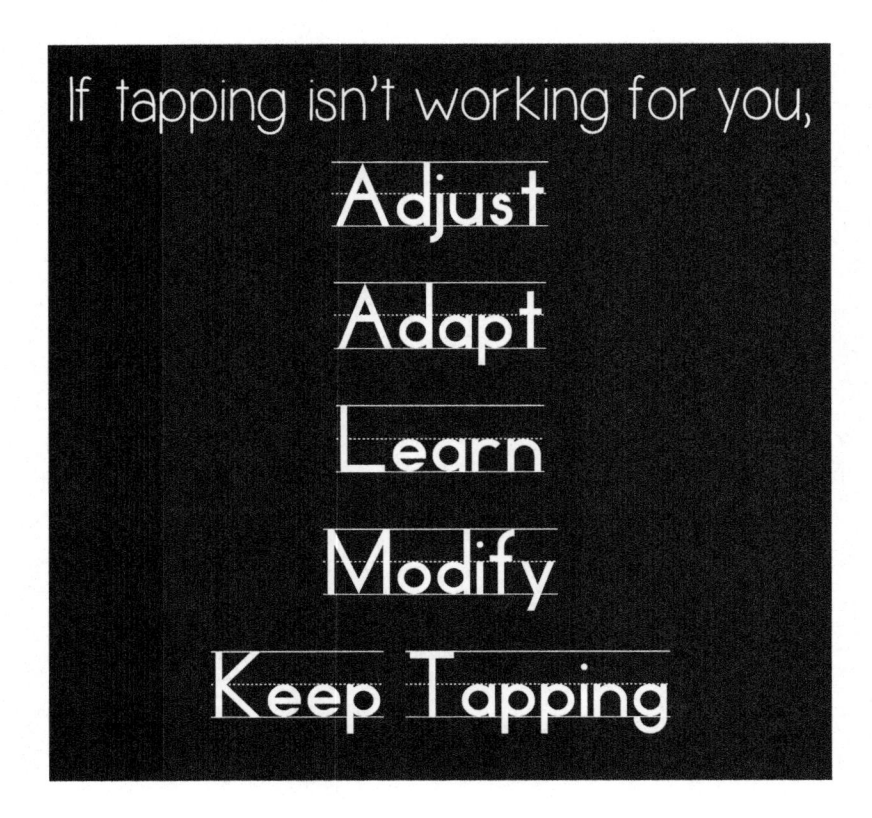

If tapping isn't working for you,

Adjust

Adapt

Learn

Modify

Keep Tapping

Chapter 17
What to Do If an EFT Tapping Statement Does Not Clear

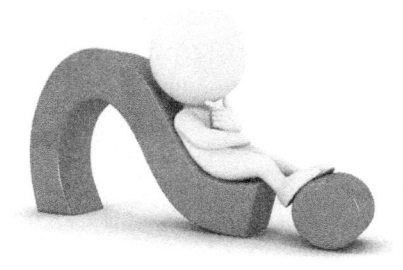

When a statement might not clear, turn the statement into a question. If the statement, "It's not okay for me to be powerful," didn't clear, **turn the tapping statement into a question:** "Why isn't it okay for me to be powerful?"

The answer might be:

* Powerful people are ruthless and heartless.
* I am afraid of being powerful.
* Being powerful would change me for the worse.
* Power corrupts.
* People would laugh at me if I tried being powerful.
* I might be called aggressive if I tried being powerful.
* I don't have the abilities, skills, or qualities to be powerful.
* Powerful people are thoughtless and self-centered.

With these beliefs, it might not be okay or safe to be powerful or even explore the idea of being powerful. The statements above are tapping statements. Tap the answer to the question.

After tapping the answer(s) to the question, revisit the original statement that did not clear. Most likely, it will now be cleared, and you will be able to take a full, deep, and complete breath.

If not, ask more questions and tap the answers. What we tapped, cleared. If you are not able to take a deep breath after tapping, the bottom-line cause has not been found yet. Keep asking questions and tapping until the underlying cause has been discovered and healed.

Do I Keep Tapping the Same Statement If It Doesn't Clear?

Tapping round after round after round, repeating the same statement over and over again as we tap does not ensure success.

For example: we tapped, "It is not okay or safe for me to be wealthy." It did not clear after one round of EFT Tapping. We truly want to be wealthy, so we continue to tap, round after round and the statement will not clear. We must dig deeper into other beliefs we have.

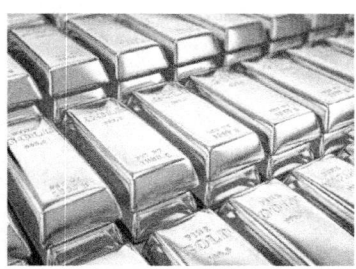

What other beliefs might we have about money?

* It is not okay for me to have more than others.
* People might try to manipulate me for my money.
* My spending might get out of control.
* Others would think I am arrogant and better than them if I
  had money.

With beliefs such as these, it might not be okay or safe to be wealthy. Rather than tapping round after round after round of the same statement, turn the statement into a question and tap the answers. "Well, why would it not be okay or safe for me to be wealthy?"

The answer you might discover is:

* I do not have the tools and skills to manage money.
* I have to work hard for my money.
* It is too much stress to maintain a wealthy lifestyle.
* The economy is too volatile and unpredictable. I might end
  up losing my wealth.

Once you uncover the additional beliefs and tap those statements, the previous statement(s) that did not clear most likely will have cleared.

AN ISSUE KEEPS SHOWING UP IN MY LIFE AFTER TAPPING

"I processed the issue I had, and I am not any better. Why?"

When we tap and process an issue, and the issue persists, it is not the process that did not work; it is the issue we processed. The correct CAUSE was not processed.

For instance, we resist change and often say, "I know I need to change, but..."

* Is the issue our resistance to change, or do we lack something to move toward?

* We process being stuck in the past, but the real issue might be that we have nothing to move forward to in the future.

* Maybe it is about our lack of goals or not having the skills to fulfill a goal.

* Maybe it is our lack of dreams and believing this is the best our life will ever be.

For instance, we may feel it is selfish to put ourselves and our needs first.

* Something bad will happen to those we love if we do not put them first.

* Others might call me selfish if I take care of my needs before theirs.

So, we process our selfishness. We process what others might say or think if we put ourselves first. Maybe the issue is not what others will think and say. Maybe the issue is us. Maybe we are just not that important to ourselves. Maybe the issue is self-love, self-respect, and self-worth.

When we process, and the same issue persists,
it is not the process that did not work.
It is the issue we processed

For example, our eating is out of control. So, we process this issue, but our eating remains out of control. Maybe the issue is not about our eating being out of control.

* Maybe the issue is about stress or lack of self-confidence or anger, fear, and/or apathy that result in overeating.

* Maybe the issue is the lack of control we feel we have in our life.

* Maybe our out-of-control eating is a symptom that our life is out of balance.

If we process and the issue seems to persist, look at the issue again, but from a different perspective. Flip it around. Look at it from the opposite perspective.

Process this new perspective.

* It might be about the future, not the past.

* It might be about our self-respect rather than someone else's respect for us.

* Maybe it is a symptom of another issue.

Flip it around
Look at the issue from another perspective

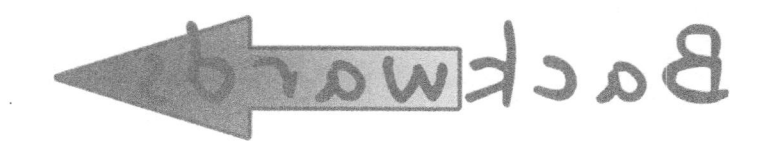

Chapter 18
Does a Negative Statement Parrot My Negative Self-Talk?

A tapping statement with the word "no" or "not" may sound like our inner critic and/or our negative self-talk. Our inner critic and negative self-talk are actually our teachers. They are letting us know the dysfunctional beliefs we need to change to advance toward health, wealth, and well-being.

Since we ignore their words of wisdom, it seems as if our inner voice is critical and negative, as if they are nagging us. The truth is this: They are pointing out what needs to be healed in order for us to be healthy, wealthy, happy, and wise!

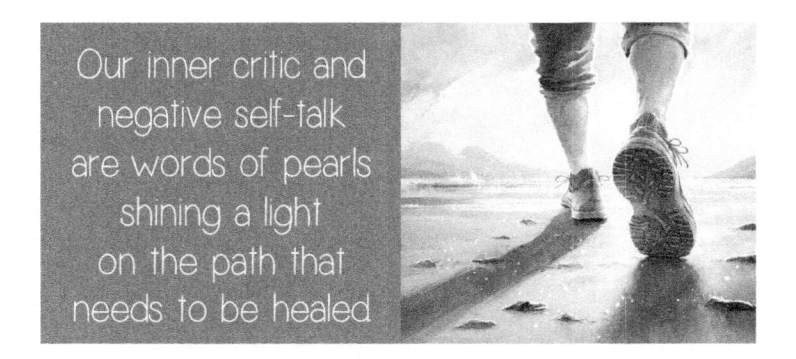

Our inner critic and negative self-talk are words of pearls shining a light on the path that needs to be healed

For example, let's say our negative self-talk goes something like this, "I will never lose the weight." What might the body be trying to tell us?

* Maybe the beliefs of being able to lose weight need to be examined and healed.

* Maybe it is about being visible and present or dealing with the anger and shame beneath the weight or about our fear of intimacy and closeness.

The body has an Infinite Wisdom. It will always gravitate toward health, peace, and joy. When we tap, we are calling forth our Truths, our Infinite Wisdom. EFT Tapping will not change our Truth. Gravity exists on Earth. Tapping will not change whether I would be affected by gravity or not.

We cannot gravitate to health, peace, wealth, and joy if we are being prevented from doing so. "Blocked energy," or energy that is not able to flow freely in the body, prevents us from gravitating to wellness, prosperity, and happiness.

Energy that is able to flow freely
will allow our bodies to heal

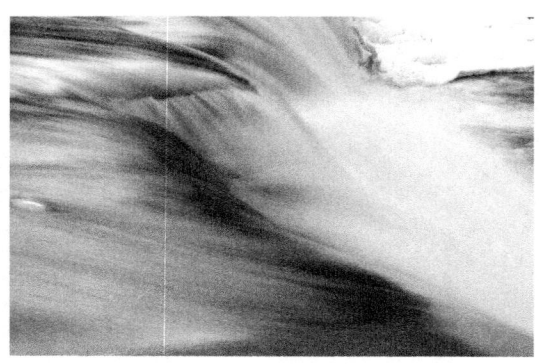

Chapter 19
Science and EFT Tapping Research

EFT has been researched in more than ten countries by over sixty investigators whose results have been published in more than twenty different peer-reviewed journals. Two leading researchers are Dawson Church, Ph.D. and David Feinstein, Ph.D.

Dr. Dawson Church, a leading expert on energy psychology and an EFT master, has gathered all the research information, and it can be found on this website: www.EFTUniverse.com.

TWO RESEARCH STUDIES

1) HARVARD MEDICAL SCHOOL STUDIES AND THE BRAIN'S STRESS RESPONSE

Studies at the Harvard Medical School reveal that tapping points along energy meridians significantly reduces activity in a part of the brain called the amygdala.

The amygdala can be thought of as the body's alarm system. When the body is experiencing trauma or fear, the amygdala is triggered, and the body is flooded with cortisol, also known as the stress hormone.

2) Dr. Dawson Church and Cortisol Reduction

Another significant study was conducted by Dr. Dawson Church. He studied the impact an hour's tapping session had on the cortisol levels of eighty-three subjects. He also measured the cortisol levels of people who received traditional talk therapy and those of a third group who received no treatment at all.

On average, for the eighty-three subjects who completed an hour tapping session, cortisol levels were reduced by 24%. Some subjects experienced a 50% reduction in cortisol levels.

The subjects who completed one hour of traditional talk therapy and those who received neither therapies (tapping or talk therapy), did not experience any significant cortisol reduction.

With hundreds of research studies, EFT Tapping is an evidence-based self-help tool that has been proven to improve our physical, mental, and emotional well-being.

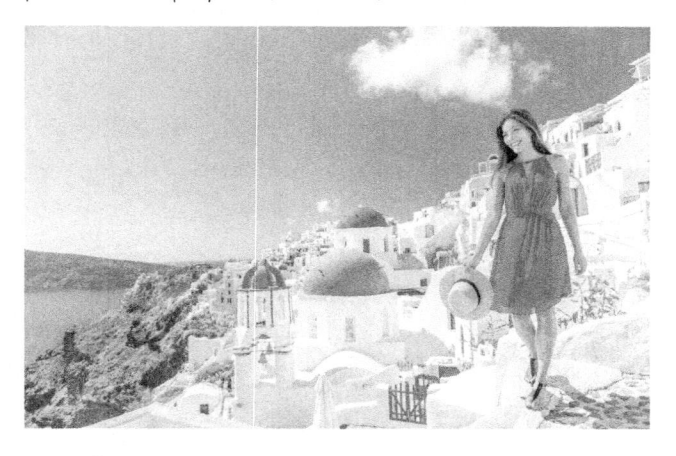

Chapter 20
Is Lowering Our Cortisol Levels Enough to Change Our Lives Permanently?

Several things can lower our cortisol (stress hormone) levels, including:

* Power posing (superman and wonder woman pose with hands on waist)
* Meditating
* Laughing
* Exercising regularly
* Listening to music
* Getting a massage
* Eliminating caffeine from our diet
* Eating a balanced, nutritious meal and eliminating processed food

Would performing any of the above activities lower our cortisol levels enough to permanently change our lives? Only if the activity eliminates dysfunctional beliefs on a subconscious level.

All of our thoughts, feelings, actions, reactions, choices, and decisions are preceded by a belief. To change our lives, dysfunctional beliefs must be eliminated.

Power posing, listening to music, or eating a balanced meal will not permanently change our lives. Exercising will help our physical body but will not delete our dysfunctional beliefs. Laughing will bring us into the present so we will not be drawn into our fears or anger, but it will not change our lives. Meditating helps us to center and balance, but it will not change our lives on a permanent basis.

To change our lives, we must recognize, acknowledge, and take ownership of what we want to change, and then delete dysfunctional emotions and beliefs on the subconscious level.

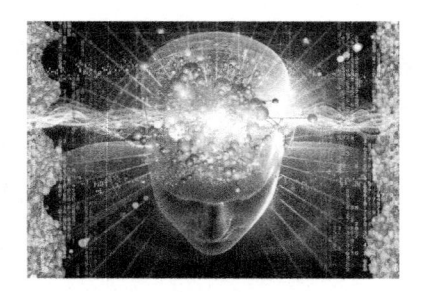

EFT Tapping will delete dysfunctional emotions and beliefs on a subconscious level if we provide the correct "instructions" to our subconscious mind. We must word the tapping statements in the subconscious' language. We must word the tapping statement so the subconscious mind hears what we want to eliminate.

Chapter 21
Tapping Affirmations

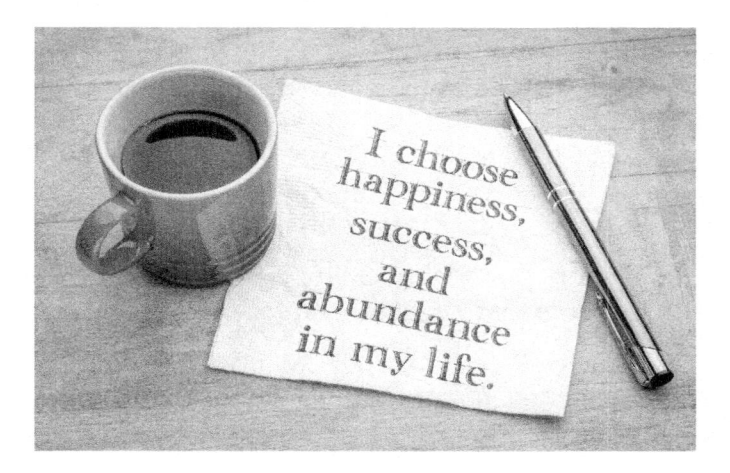

Do you repeat these affirmations?

1. I am healthy and happy.
2. Wealth is pouring into my life.
3. I radiate love and happiness.
4. I have the perfect job for me.
5. I am successful in whatever I do.

If we were to tap "I am healthy and happy now" and we are not, most likely, as we are tapping, we might think, "Yeah, right. Sure. I am healthy and happy. My life sucks. I hate my job. I am always broke. There is never enough money."

The body knows this is not true. We are not healthy and happy now. When we tap, we might have difficulty remembering what we are saying, lose focus and concentration, and/or the mind drifts.

An EFT Tapping statement is most effective **when** it matches our current belief.

The subconscious does not hear the word "No." One way of tapping affirmations and, at the same time, increase our positive outlook, is by adding the word "no" into the tapping statements.

1. I am **not** healthy and happy. Subconscious hears: I am healthy and happy.
2. Wealth is **not** pouring into my life. Subconscious hears: Wealth is pouring into my life.
3. I **do not** radiate love and happiness. Subconscious hears: I radiate love and happiness.
4. I **do not** have the perfect job for me. Subconscious hears: I have the perfect job for me.
5. I am **not** successful in whatever I do. Subconscious hears: I am successful in whatever I do.

If we repeat affirmations over and over before we clear the affirmation with EFT Tapping, it will have little effect. Repeating affirmations creates circumstances in our lives where we are confronted by our beliefs that do not align with the affirmation.

For affirmations to be most beneficial, tap the affirmation by adding a "no" to the tapping statement.

Chapter 22
Finishing Touches –
Positive Statements

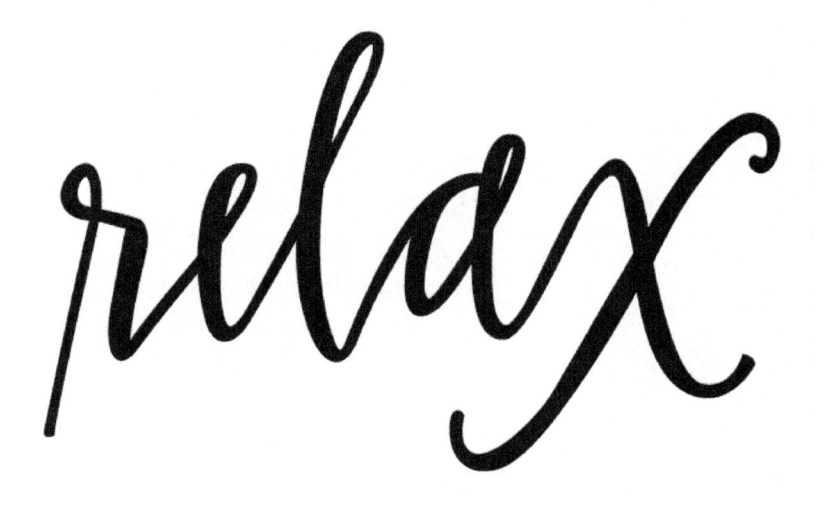

Some people like to finish their tapping with statements that are centering and calming. If this is you, then you might want to try the sixteen statements on the next page or make up those that you like. The statements can be said in any order that works for you.

Tapping Location	Statement
Eyebrow	All is well in my life.
Temple	Every day in every way I am getting better and better.
Under the Eye	I am fulfilled in every way, every day.
Under the Nose	My blessings appears in rich appropriate form with divine timing.
Under the Lips	I am an excellent steward of wealth and am blessed with great abundance.
Under the Collar-bone Knob	I take complete responsibility for everything in my life.
Under the Arm	I have all the tools, skills, and abilities to excel in my life.
Top back part of the Head	I know I will be able to handle anything that arises in my life.
Eyebrow	All my dreams, hopes, wishes, and goals are being fulfilled each and every day.
Temple	Divine love expressing through me, now draws to me new ideas.
Under the Eye	I am comfortable with my life changing.
Under the Nose	I am able to create all that I desire.
Under the Lips	I know what needs to be done and follow through to completion.
Under the Collar-bone Knob	My health is perfect in every way, physically, mentally, emotionally, and spiritually.
Under the Arm	I invite into my subconscious Archangel Raphael to heal all that needs to be forgiven, released, and redeemed. Cleanse me and free me from it now.
Top back part of the Head	The light of God surrounds me. The love of God enfolds me. The power of God protects me. The presence of God watches over and flows through me.

Chapter 23 – How to Use This Book

1. The statements are divided into sections. Read through the statements in one section. Notice if you have any reaction to the statement or feel the statement might be true for you. If so, note the number for that statement.

2. List the top seven or more statements.

3. From this list, select one and describe how it plays out in your life. It is important to recognize and identify the patterns, the consequences of having this belief, the trigger(s), and how it begins.

4. Tap the statements. Statements can be combined for scripts.

5. After tapping, review the statements to determine if you still have a reaction to any of the statements or you do not think the statement cleared. If you do, you have several options:
A) Put a "Why" before the statement. Tap the answers.
B) Keep a list of statements that do not clear. After additional tapping, return to this list to determine if the statement has cleared. Statements that still have not cleared, put a "why" before the statement and tap the answers.

6. Allow some downtime for integration and the body to heal.

7. The number of sections you do at a time will be up to you. Initially, you might want to do one section to determine if you get tired and need to have some downtime after tapping.

Chapter 24
EFT Tapping Statements 1 – 20

Those on top of the mountain did not fall there.

Marcus Washling

1. I have no life.
2. I knowingly lie.
3. I resist change.
4. I lack discipline.
5. I quit before I fail.
6. I am never wrong.
7. I stretch the truth.
8. I am stuck in a rut.
9. I stuff my feelings.
10. I'm quick to judge.
11. I am a couch potato.
12. I have to be perfect.
13. I feel small and weak.
14. Life is passing me by.
15. I am a people pleaser.
16. I jump to conclusions.
17. I am easily distracted.
18. My life lacks structure.
19. I need to be in control.
20. I am not smart enough.

Journaling for Statements 1 – 20

Loser's visualize the penalties of failure.
Winners visualize the rewards of success.

Dr. Rob Gilbert

1. From the tapping statements in this section, tap the top seven statements that you thought or felt applied to you:

1.

2.

3.

4.

5.

6.

7.

2. From this list above, select one and describe how it plays out in your life. Give an example. It is important to recognize and identify the pattern, triggers, how it begins, how has it benefited and harmed you? For instance, will you always be a loser? What makes you a loser? What would make you a winner? Are you willing to do the work being a winner requires?

EFT Tapping Statements 21 - 40

A kite flies best when the wind blows in one direction and the string pulls from another.

Henry Ford

21. I have to play my life small.
22. I will never get what I want.
23. I don't go after what I want.
24. What I want doesn't matter.
25. I hide my feelings of shame.
26. I am stupid, dumb, and ugly.
27. It's difficult to make friends.
28. I never let anyone get close.
29. Most of life is disappointing.
30. I will never amount to much.
31. I am inadequate and broken.
32. I am not in charge of my life.
33. Compliments embarrass me.
34. I am controlled by my anger.
35. I am afraid of looking foolish.
36. I hit burnout a long time ago.
37. I am stupid and incompetent.
38. I am plagued with self-doubt.
39. My faults are many and huge.
40. I overanalyze things to death.

Journaling for Statements 21 – 40

If there is a most likely to succeed, I was the least.

Michael Jordan

1. From the tapping statements in this section, tap the top seven statements that you thought or felt applied to you:

1.

2.

3.

4.

5.

6.

7.

2. From this list above, select one and describe how it plays out in your life. Give an example. It is important to recognize and identify the pattern, triggers, how it begins, how has it benefited and harmed you? For instance, are you plagues with self-doubt? Is this about possibly failing at achieving a task and thus are fearful to move forward? Or are you so comfortable in your comfort zone you don't want to make the effort stepping outside your comfort zone would require?

EFT Tapping Statements 41 – 60

There are no secrets to success. It is the result
of preparation, hard work, and learning from failure

Colin Powell

41. I don't fit in anywhere.

42. I exaggerate my worth.

43. I have to win at all cost.

44. I need other's approval.

45. I have no need of goals.

46. My goals never happen.

47. I live beyond my means.

48. I get discouraged easily.

49. I don't believe in myself.

50. No one understands me.

51. I don't trust my instincts.

52. I need people to like me.

53. I make sarcastic remarks.

54. I eat to fill the loneliness.

55. Inner peace is an illusion.

56. I tolerate the intolerable.

57. I'm defective, full of flaws.

58. I am reluctant to set goals.

59. I deny my emotional needs.

60. I sabotage my own success.

Journaling for Statements 41 – 60

I will always have a shadow whenever I step into the light.

Tessa Cason

1. From the tapping statements in this section, tap the top seven statements that you thought or felt applied to you:

1.

2.

3.

4.

5.

6.

7.

2. From this list above, select one and describe how it plays out in your life. Give an example. It is important to recognize and identify the pattern, triggers, how it begins, how has it benefited and harmed you? For instance, do you eat to fill the loneliness? Has food become your best friend? Is it easier to eat rather than to move out of your comfort zone and build friendships?

EFT Tapping Statements 61 – 80

You can make a fresh start any moment you choose. This thing we call "failure" is not the falling down, but the staying down.

Mary Pickford

61. I avoid confrontation at all cost.
62. Life is unfair, abusive, and cruel.
63. I stay in unhealthy relationships.
64. I can't bounce back after defeat.
65. I overreact to defeat and failure.
66. I fight with others for no reason.
67. I complicate the simplest things.
68. I secretly hope other people fail.
69. I have no clue what I want in life.
70. I have to give up me to be loved.
71. I have difficulty asserting myself.
72. It is difficult for me to be myself.
73. I lie even when it isn't necessary.
74. I will not give up my addiction(s).
75. I am not qualified to do anything.
76. I pick fights to push people away.
77. I have difficulty completing tasks.
78. I overindulge in escapist activities.
79. I spot rejection where none exists.
80. I need to be the center of attention.

Journaling for Statements 61 – 80

Show me someone who has done something worthwhile and I will show you someone who has overcome adversity.

Lou Holtz

1. From the tapping statements in this section, tap the top seven statements that you thought or felt applied to you:

1.

2.

3.

4.

5.

6.

7.

2. From this list above, select one and describe how it plays out in your life. Give an example. It is important to recognize and identify the pattern, triggers, how it begins, how has it benefited and harmed you? For instance, do you complicate the simplest things? If so, does something have to be complicated to be worthwhile doing? Does this make you feel more competent if you are able to handle something complicated? Is this about what others will think? Will others think you more capable if you are able to successfully handle complex tasks?

EFT Tapping Statements 81 – 100

Every thought is a seed If you plant crab apples,
don't count on harvesting Golden Delicious.

Bill Meyer

81. I will never achieve my goals.
82. I complaint and criticize a lot.
83. I don't do well with deadlines.
84. I lack motivation to do my life.
85. I don't live up to my potential.
86. I am oversensitive to criticism.
87. I give up after the first defeat.
88. No one wants to be my friend.
89. Nothing will help my situation.
90. I am a victim of circumstances.
91. No one really understands me.
92. I'm defective, damaged goods.
93. I argue for the sake of arguing.
94. I am easily taken advantage of.
95. I am not worthy of what I want.
96. I have a tendency to overreact.
97. I have no choice but to say yes.
98. Others make my life miserable.
99. I feel lost, confused, and afraid.
100. My behavior is self-destructive.

Journaling for Statements 81 – 100

The first and greatest form of courage is the courage to take responsible for your own life. Like it or not, you alone are responsible for the person you are today, the state of your heart, and the shape of your life. You can point your finger 'til the cows come home, but at the end of the day, the buck stops with you.

Margie Warrell

1. From the tapping statements in this section, tap the top seven statements that you thought or felt applied to you:

1.

2.

3.

4.

5.

6.

7.

2. From this list above, select one and describe how it plays out in your life. Give an example. It is important to recognize and identify the pattern, triggers, how it begins, how has it benefited and harmed you? For instance,do you live up to your potential? If not, is this an issue of apathy, fear, anxiety, goal setting, power, establishing a plan to fulfill your goals, and/or lack of direction?

EFT Tapping Statements 101 – 120

The cave you fear to enter
holds the treasure you seek.

Joseph Campbell

101. I can't find any enjoyment in my life.
102. I don't know how to reinvent myself.
103. I find it difficult to enjoy what I have.
104. I bully others to hide my insecurities.
105. Bad things will happen if I am happy.
106. Every setback is major drama for me.
107. I avoid the spotlight or any attention.
108. My dreams will never become reality.
109. I'm not sure what will make me happy.
110. I am unable to maintain a relationship.
111. I blame others for my problems in life.
112. I have an excessive need for approval.
113. I knowingly hurt others and/or myself.
114. I freeze up when I need to take action.
115. I manipulate others to get what I want.
116. I don't have a clue what my values are.
117. I worry about how others perceive me.
118. I avoid new people and new situations.
119. I live my life in a state of constant fear.
120. I cannot depend on anyone but myself.

Journaling for Statements 101 – 120

To every person there comes that special moment when
he is tapped on the shoulder to do a very special thing unique
to them. What a tragedy if that moment finds them
unprepared for the work that would be their finest hour.

Winston Churchill

1. From the tapping statements in this section, tap the top
seven statements that you thought or felt applied to you:

1.

2.

3.

4.

5.

6.

7.

2. From this list above, select one and describe how it plays
out in your life. Give an example. It is important to recognize
and identify the pattern, triggers, how it begins, how has it
benefited and harmed you? For instance, is it easier to blame
others for your lack of action? Do you know the action that is
required? Do you have the skills needed that the action
would require? Or is it easier to blame someone else for your
lack of knowledge and skill?

EFT Tapping Statements 121 – 140

Progress always involves risk. You can not steal
second base and keep your foot on first.

Frederick Wilcox

121. I make mountains out of molehills.

122. I'm detached from life and my life.

123. I berate myself if I make a mistake.

124. I cannot accept the flaws in myself.

125. My worst fears are always realized.

126. I blame others for my unhappiness.

127. I hate me and everything about me.

128. I brood about my current problems.

129. I feel worse when things get better.

130. I can be very judgmental and mean.

131. I am reluctant to plan for my future.

132. I will do anything to avoid rejection.

133. I am not smart, talented, or capable.

134. Others ridicule and make fun of me.

135. I waste time with meaningless tasks.

136. Everything must revolve around me.

137. I am not accountable or responsible.

138. I crave approval, attention, and love.

139. I turn every crisis into a catastrophe.

140. It is too scary getting close to others.

Journaling for Statements 121 – 140

Our suffering comes from wanting things to be
different. When we stop that, our suffering stops. We
can want things. It is the needing that must stop.

Wayne Dyer

1. From the tapping statements in this section, tap the top
seven statements that you thought or felt applied to you:

1.

2.

3.

4.

5.

6.

7.

2. From this list above, select one and describe how it plays
out in your life. Give an example. It is important to recognize
and identify the pattern, triggers, how it begins, how has it
benefited and harmed you? For instance, do you have difficulty finding success in your failures? Is this about needing to
be perfect, not knowing how to learn life's lessons, or a reason to find fault with yourself?

EFT Tapping Statements 141 – 160

We are all faced with a series of great opportunities brilliantly disguised as unsolvable problems.

John W. Gardner

141. I don't know how to give up my excuses.
142. I am a victim of other people's decisions.
143. I constantly feel drained and exhausted.
144. Nothing I do will ever make a difference.
145. I am overwhelmed with the task of living.
146. I am totally consumed by fear and doubt.
147. I feel powerless around powerful people.
148. I shouldn't have to tell other what I need.
149. I avoid confrontation by being agreeable.
150. I'm waiting for those in my life to change.
151. I blame others for not fulfilling my needs.
152. I retell my woes to anyone that will listen.
153. I obsess over the littlest, stupidest things.
154. No one is interested in what I have to say.
155. I get anxious when things start to go well.
156. I don't feel a part of the world around me.
157. People don't give me the credit I deserve.
158. I anticipate negative results and reactions.
159. I need medication to keep me functioning.
160. I don't have the same choices others have.

Journaling for Statements 141 – 160

Denial is pushing something out of your awareness.
Anything you hide in the basement has a way of burrowing
under the house and showing up on the front lawn.

Howard Sasportas

1. From the tapping statements in this section, tap the top seven statements that you thought or felt applied to you:

1.

2.

3.

4.

5.

6.

7.

2. From this list above, select one and describe how it plays out in your life. Give an example. It is important to recognize and identify the pattern, triggers, how it begins, how has it benefited and harmed you? For instance, do you avoid confrontations by being agreeable? Do you know your point of view? Do you know how to express your ideas when they might be different than others? Do you fear rejection if you express ideas that are different?

EFT Tapping Statements 161 – 180

*Action without planning is fatal
but planning without action is futile.*

Tracie Van Eimeren

161. I have difficulty asking for what I want.
162. I apologize even when it's not my fault.
163. I push people away who could help me.
164. I would be elated if I could be invisible.
165. There is nothing I am passionate about.
166. I put off today what I can do tomorrow.
167. I am weak, defenseless, and vulnerable.
168. I don't know how to change my actions.
169. I act impulsively in important situations.
170. I put things off or never get them done.
171. I take on more than I am able to handle.
172. I drag myself out of bed every morning.
173. I have difficulty accepting compliments.
174. I am overly critical of myself and others.
175. I am reluctant to share my true feelings.
176. I never seem to be on time for anything.
177. I have a defeatist attitude and mentality.
178. I am not aware of my options or choices.
179. I am jealous of everyone and everything.
180. I feel empty, disappointed, and betrayed.

Journaling for Statements 161 – 180

In the middle of difficulty lies opportunity.

Albert Einstein

1. From the tapping statements in this section, tap the top seven statements that you thought or felt applied to you:

1.

2.

3.

4.

5.

6.

7.

2. From this list above, select one and describe how it plays out in your life. Give an example. It is important to recognize and identify the pattern, triggers, how it begins, how has it benefited and harmed you? For instance, there is nothing you are passionate about. Is this to avoid disappointment if you "fail" at something you are passionate about? Is this about fear that you might not have the talents, skills, and abilities that your passion would require? Or is it easier to shut down emotional and pretend you are not passionate about anything?

EFT Tapping Statements 181 – 200

We are always trying to move out of the darkness,
when all we have to do is turn on the light.

Steve Potter

181. I sacrifice my needs for the sake of others.
182. I berate myself if I make the wrong choice.
183. I can't commit to anything wholeheartedly.
184. I lack compassion for others and/or myself.
185. I have been hurt, ignored, and browbeaten.
186. I don't know how to move beyond my grief.
187. It is hopeless that my life will ever be good.
188. I get wrapped up in the problems of others.
189. I cannot depend or trust anyone but myself.
190. I end relationships before I can be rejected.
191. I'm afraid of being rejected and abandoned.
192. I act cruelly toward the people I care about.
193. I am constantly comparing myself to others.
194. I can't live up to others' expectations of me.
195. I have difficulty concentrating and focusing.
196. I overindulge in alcohol, drugs, and/or food.
197. I am insensitive to everything and everyone.
198. There are some people that easily annoy me.
199. I don't expect good things to happen for me.
200. I am dependent, incapable, and incompetent.

Journaling for Statements 181 – 200

The greatest thing is, at any moment, to be willing to give up who you are in order to become all that you can become.

Max de Pree

1. From the tapping statements in this section, tap the top seven statements that you thought or felt applied to you:

1.

2.

3.

4.

5.

6.

7.

2. From this list above, select one and describe how it plays out in your life. Give an example. It is important to recognize and identify the pattern, triggers, how it begins, how has it benefited and harmed you? For instance, are you still waiting for things to happen? Who's in control? The person or circumstances you are waiting to make something happen for you? What would be required of you to take the action necessary for something to happen? Do you have the courage to make things happen for yourself?

EFT Tapping Statements 201 – 220

*Failure is the opportunity to
begin again more intelligently.*

Henry Ford

201. I am constantly wringing my hands in worry.
202. I would be ridiculed if I shared my emotions.
203. I don't know how to move beyond my anger.
204. I am having difficulty getting on with my life.
205. I am afraid of authority and authority figures.
206. I miss important meetings and appointments.
207. I constantly question my abilities and talents.
208. I have difficulty expressing negative feelings.
209. My dreams and desires will never be fulfilled.
210. Those that love me should know what I need.
211. I have a fear of performing or doing anything.
212. I don't know how to move beyond my regrets.
213. I give up what I want to accommodate others.
214. Obstacles weaken my resolve and motivation.
215. I am weak, helpless, needy, and/or frightened.
216. I attract the wrong type of people into my life.
217. I try to control everything that happens to me.
218. I compare myself to others and come up short.
219. I test everyone for evidence that they love me.
220. I have been harassed, degraded, and neglected.

Journaling for Statements 201 – 220

The road to success has many tempting parking places

Steve Potter

1. From the tapping statements in this section, tap the top seven statements that you thought or felt applied to you:

1.

2.

3.

4.

5.

6.

7.

2. From this list above, select one and describe how it plays out in your life. Give an example. It is important to recognize and identify the pattern, triggers, how it begins, how has it benefited and harmed you? For instance, do you try to control everything that happens to you? Is this about your inability to be flexible, your insecurities, and/or wanting to appear powerful?

EFT Tapping Statements 221 – 240

one asks for success and prepares for failure,
one will get the situation they prepared for.

Florence Scovel Shinn

221. I have an emptiness that I don't know how to fill.
222. My negative self has the dominant role in my life.
223. I don't know how to find what's missing in my life.
224. Praise and compliments make me uncomfortable.
225. I'm not supposed to be happy or show happiness.
226. It is not okay/safe to show tears or be vulnerable.
227. I base my behavior on what I believe others want.
228. I'm too stuck in the past to move into the present.
229. I make myself small so others can be comfortable.
230. I put myself down before others have a chance to.
231. I don't know why bad things always happen to me.
232. I push other's hot buttons when I am mad at them.
233. I don't take responsibility for myself or my actions.
234. I will do anything not to hurt or disappoint anyone.
235. I have made choices that didn't work out very well.
236. I tell white lies to make others feel good about me.
237. I let my insecurities interfere with my relationships.
238. Doing anything new is too frightening for me to do.
239. I am overly concerned about the opinions of others.
240. I take responsibility for everything that goes wrong.

Journaling for Statements 221 – 240

Hiding in my room, safe within my womb, I
touch no one and no one touches me. I am a
rock, I am an island And a rock feels no pain;
And an island never cries.

Paul Simon, From song I Am a Rock

1. From the tapping statements in this section, tap the top
seven statements that you thought or felt applied to you:

1.

2.

3.

4.

5.

6.

7.

2. From this list above, select one and describe how it plays
out in your life. Give an example. It is important to recognize
and identify the pattern, triggers, how it begins, how has it
benefited and harmed you? For instance, do you make yourself small so others can be comfortable? Is this about your or
them? Is this about your belonging need and afraid if you
aren't small that need won't be fulfilled? Or is this about others might fault with you if you were noticed?

EFT Tapping Statements 241 – 260

The worst loneliness is to not
be comfortable with yourself.

Mark Twain

241. I freak out when I am faced with the unknown.

242. I don't know how to overcome my insecurities.

243. I spend the majority of my life on the sidelines.

244. I always put others' needs first before my own.

245. I am waiting for a disaster to strike at any time.

246. I don't know how to move beyond my self-pity.

247. My favorite topic of discussion is my problems.

248. I can become extremely irritable and impatient.

249. I use food as a substitute for friends and family.

250. It would be arrogant of me to think I had worth.

251. I have difficulty confronting stressful situations.

252. I don't seem to be able to get myself organized.

253. I blame outside circumstances for my problems.

254. I say hurtful things to people I really care about.

255. I feel alone even when I'm around other people.

256. I am not in control of the direction my life takes.

257. I can't stand up for myself even when I am right.

258. It is uncomfortable for me to ask others for help.

259. I am having trouble moving pass my resentment.

260. I have an excuse for everything that goes wrong.

Journaling for Statements 241 – 260

*Every human being on this earth is born with
the tragedy that they have to grow up. A lot
of people do not have the courage to do it.*

Helen Hayes

1. From the tapping statements in this section, tap the top seven statements that you thought or felt applied to you:

1.

2.

3.

4.

5.

6.

7.

2. From this list above, select one and describe how it plays out in your life. Give an example. It is important to recognize and identify the pattern, triggers, how it begins, how has it benefited and harmed you? For instance, would it be arrogant of you to think you had worth? What does inner confidence, authentic power, and rock solid serenity look like?

EFT Tapping Statements 261 – 280

Pain is inevitable.
Suffering is optional.

Dr. H. White

261. I'm constantly anxious that I'll do something wrong.
262. I am always blamed for everything that goes wrong.
263. I need and want instant and immediate gratification.
264. My burdens are too overwhelming for me to handle.
265. I'm quick to make up my mind and slow to change it.
266. No one will ever love me the way I need to be loved.
267. I respond negatively to anyone that offers a solution.
268. I avoid challenges, new tasks, and new opportunities.
269. There is no one and nothing that is going to help me.
270. I don't allow myself to grieve, be sad, or feel my pain.
271. I am annoyed when someone doesn't take my advice.
272. I am so busy helping others I have no time for myself.
273. I am delicate and need to be handled with great care.
274. I don't seem to be able to stop the defeatist thoughts.
275. I am not able to enjoy things that should be enjoyable.
276. Something holds me back from going full steam ahead.
277. I wait for everything to be perfect before taking action.
278. I have unrealistic expectations for myself and/or others.
279. My moods are subject to the whims and words of others.
280. There is a deep void in me that always needs to be filled.

Journaling for Statements 261 – 280

There is no traffic jam on the extra mile.

Business axiom

1. From the tapping statements in this section, tap the top seven statements that you thought or felt applied to you:

1.

2.

3.

4.

5.

6.

7.

2. From this list above, select one and describe how it plays out in your life. Give an example. It is important to recognize and identify the pattern, triggers, how it begins, how has it benefited and harmed you? For instance, do you wait for everything to be perfect before taking action? If so, are you still waiting? What would happen if you took action before everything was perfect? Are you afraid you might fail? Do you know how to learn from your failures? Do you know how to make lemonade out of lemons? Add sugar...

EFT Tapping Statements 281 – 300

I will love the light for it shows me the way, yet I will endure the darkness because it shows me the stars

Og Mandino

281. I have a million excuses for my lack of accomplishments.
282. I am jealous and envious of others that have what I want.
283. I am suspicious of anything good that happens in my life.
284. I know what needs to be done and still don't do anything.
285. I don't know what to say when someone compliments me.
286. I'm caught up in a loop of self-destruct and self-sabotage.
287. I avoid conflict by walking away and ignoring the problem.
288. I'm glued to TV from the time I get home until I go to bed.
289. I'm doomed to a life of failure, misery, and disappointment.
290. I lack motivation to do pretty much everything and anything.
291. I am helpless to do anything to improve the quality of my life.
292. I am intimidated by those who are more competent than I am.
293. I just don't seem to be able to generate a passion for anything.
294. I'm hesitant to give my opinion for fear someone will not like it.
295. I have to be the one to make it happen if anything is to happen.

296. I have difficulty tolerating imperfection in myself and/or others.
297. I wait for the other shoe to drop when something good happens.
298. I shy away from organizing, planning, and preparing for my future.
299. I don't do the things that would make me feel healthier and happier.
300. I hide my head in the sand hoping that problems will resolve themselves.

Journaling for Statements 281 – 300

Critics hang around and wait for others to make mistakes.
The real doers of the world have no time for criticizing others.
They are too busy doing, making mistakes, improving, making
progress. They are committed to themselves, their growth, their lives.

Dr. Wayne Dyer

1. From the tapping statements in this section, tap the top seven statements that you thought or felt applied to you:

1.

2.

3.

4.

5.

6.

7.

2. From this list above, select one and describe how it plays out in your life. Give an example. It is important to recognize and identify the pattern, triggers, how it begins, how has it benefited and harmed you? For instance, are you intimidated by those who are more competent than you are? Usually, lack of action follows intimidation. What would be needed for you to be inspired instead of intimidated?

New Product Launching Fall 2023

Tessa created a new series call *Awaken, Emerge, Become* to provide a guide for a seeker to find their own insights and ah-ha wisdom. The series includes a book, card deck, journal, and Workbook and work in tandem with each other.

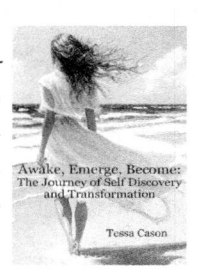

The book, *Awaken, Emerge, Become: The Journey of Self-Reflection and Transformation* is a step-by-step guide from self discovery to transformation. It includes many of the tools, techniques, and methods she learned from some remarkable teachers.

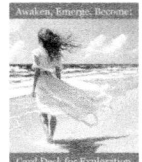

The sixty card deck, *Awaken, Emerge, Become: Card Deck of Exploration* is a fun tool to aid in finding answers, discover new insights, and might provide new awarenesses for the inquisitive.

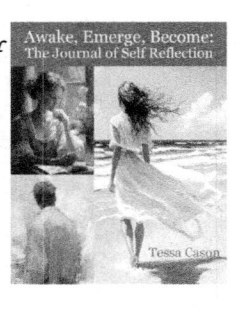

Awaken, Emerge, Become: The Journal of Self-reflection is a series of questions to help a seeker discern their truths. The intent of the journal is to assist you in finding your ah-ha wisdom, answers to the challenges you currently are facing, and possible paths to healing physically, mentally, emotionally, and spiritually.

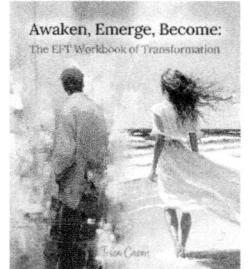

Awaken, Emerge, Become: The EFT Workbook for Transformation is a step-by-step guide to becoming the highest potential of ourselves.

Books by Tessa Cason

200 EFT Tapping Statements for Wealth
240 EFT Tapping Statements for Fear
300 EFT Tapping Statements for Healing the Self
300 EFT Tapping Statements for Dealing with Obnoxious People
300 EFT Tapping Statements for Intuition
300 EFT Tapping Statements for Self-defeating Behaviors,
Victim, Self-pity
340 EFT Tapping Statements for Healing From the Loss
of a Loved One
400 EFT Tapping Statements for Being a Champion
400 EFT Tapping Statements for Being Empowered
and Successful
400 EFT Tapping Statements for Dealing with Emotions
400 EFT Tapping Statements for Dreams to Reality
400 EFT Tapping Statements for My Thyroid Story
500 EFT Tapping Statements for Moving Out of Survival
700 EFT Tapping Statements for Weight, Emotional Eating,
and Food Cravings
All Things EFT Tapping Manual
Emotional Significance of Human Body Parts
Muscle Testing – Obstacles and Helpful Hints

EFT TAPPING STATEMENTS FOR:
A Broken Heart, Abandonment, Anger, Depression,
Grief, Emotional Healing
Anxiety, Fear, Anger, Self Pity, Change
Champion, Success, Personal Power, Self Confidence,
Leader/Role Model
Prosperity, Survival, Courage, Personal Power, Success
PTSD, Disempowered, Survival, Fear, Anger
Weight & Food Cravings, Anger, Grief, Not Good Enough,
Failure

Printed in Great Britain
by Amazon

35831271R00076